Managing Everyday Problems

THOMAS A. BRIGHAM
Washington State University

THE GUILFORD PRESS
New York   London

© 1989 The Guilford Press
A Division of Guilford Publications, Inc.
72 Spring Street, New York, NY 10012

Printed in the United States of America

Last digit is print number: 9 8 7 6 5 4 3 2 1

ISBN 0-89862-508-4

Contents

An Introduction for the Student

As humans, we often wonder why things happen. Sometimes our questions are about physical things that happen to us. Why did the car break down just before my big date? Or, why did I catch a cold during spring vacation and have to stay home while everyone else was having fun? Sometimes we wonder about our own behavior or that of other people. For instance, Why did I get mad and yell at my mother? Why is Cathy always rude to me? Why does George act so immaturely? Why do I always seem to put my foot in my mouth when talking to girls/boys?

There are often times when we would like to change our behavior or how other people act toward us. Using the previous problems as examples, what can I do so that I don't yell at my mom? How can I get Cathy to be nice to me? How can I help George act more maturely? What can I do to become better at talking to girls/boys? It is possible to give many other examples of the problems of being a young person. It is often difficult to find someone to talk to about these problems. Adults (parents, teachers) often don't seem to understand, and your friends are often as confused by the problems as you are.

This manual was developed to provide some information about why people act the way they do and how you might be able to change your own behavior. The book provides some basic information and suggestions, but it won't solve everything. It is meant to help you solve everyday problems. But if you are worried about a serious problem, ask someone for help. A basic principle of problem solving is to use all of the resources available to you. Parents, teachers, counselors, and other adults can all be sources of information and help. The first step in solving a difficult problem is to seek help.

Many people contributed to the development of this manual. They participated in similar courses and told us what was useful, and what was irrelevant or phoney. They also made useful suggestions on how to change the manual. My own children, Jeremy and Christy, also provided valuable help by trying out the experiments, reading the units, and honestly telling me what was the matter with them. Occasionally, I thought they could have chosen better terms than "stupid" or "dumb" but these comments clearly let me know when something was poorly written. There probably is still material in the book that you may consider useless or—even worse—boring. If you have suggestions for change, tell your instructor or write to me.

The manual begins with some basic ideas. You may wonder why you should learn them, but remember that in order to perform complex skills, you must master the basics first. For example, the young person who wants to make the basketball team must first spend many long and often boring hours practicing dribbling, shooting, and passing. This practice is not as interesting or exciting as playing in the game, but it must be done to play well in the game.

Most lessons contain a study guide. You should first read the lesson carefully and then fill in the answers to the study-guide questions. Answering these questions will tell you how well you understand the lesson. After completing the study guides, you will discuss them in class, and you may do other exercises. To get the most out of the discussions and exercises, you must work hard on your own to master the material.

We hope you find the ideas and procedures described in the manual interesting and useful. Good luck!

I

PRINCIPLES AND PROCEDURES OF BEHAVIOR ANALYSIS

Science plays a preeminent role in influencing our world now, but this has not always been the case. Although it is possible to find elements of science or scientific technique in the records of early civilizations, it was not until the end of the 17th century that the procedures of measurement, experiment, and reasoning that we call science systematically emerged. In the 3 centuries or so since the publication of Newton's *Principia* in 1687, our knowledge of the universe and our ability to create new forms of knowledge has increased at an accelerating rate. In fact, our world is so profoundly different from the prescientific one that comparisons are impossible. What factors lead to the development of science and its ability to produce such powerful knowledge? Briefly, there appear to be three crucial elements shared by the various scientific disciplines. They are:

1. The development of objective methods for defining and measuring variables or phenomena
2. A reliance on empirical or inductive reasoning for the development of laws
3. The evolution of an appropriate experimental method for gathering evidence.[1]

These terms and phrases seem very abstract, but the role that each plays in a science is discussed here within the context of our study of psychology.

1. See B. Russell (1931). *The scientific outlook*. New York: W. W. Norton. pp. 13–70.

UNIT 1

Measurement and Definition of Behavior

Psychology is a science that studies the behavior of animals and humans, both children and adults. Although psychology has now established itself as a scientific discipline, it has not done so easily. The problem has been learning how to apply scientific procedures to understanding human behavior. For instance, when chemists and physicists do experiments, such as mixing two parts of hydrogen and one part oxygen under the proper conditions, they get water every time (it is very orderly). For psychologists, it is never simple to do experiments and analyze the results. This is because two people rarely, if ever, behave in the same manner, nor does one person respond to the same situation in exactly the same way. This is one of the primary reasons why psychology began to develop as a science at a much later date than physics or chemistry. Nonetheless, it is possible to conduct orderly and systematic experiments and studies in psychology by clearly defining the events (what the person or animal is doing) to be studied so that the consistent ways that different animals or people act can be measured.

In psychology, as in other sciences, the development of methods for observing and measuring events was the first step in the evolution of the discipline as a science. The initial focus in psychological measurement was on objectively defining the behavior or response in question. What is behavior? What are some examples of behavior? Is talking a behavior? Is crying a behavior? Is walking a behavior? Yes, they are behaviors of a certain type: They are all directly *observable*. These observable behaviors are called *overt behaviors*.

There are also behaviors that are not observable. For instance, you may be thinking right now about what you are going to do later. Is thinking a behavior? It is, but it is different from overt behaviors because we cannot see it. Behaviors such as thinking are therefore called *covert* or unobservable.

Psychologists study both overt and covert behavior. There are, however, quite a few problems related to finding out about covert behavior. For example, if you ask people to talk about what they are thinking or feeling or what they remember about their childhoods, most people have a great deal of trouble describing their feelings, others may forget their experiences and reactions, and some may be too embarrassed to tell someone else their thoughts. As a consequence, studies using such inconsistent or unreliable information often produced results that were confusing and contradictory. For those reasons, we focus our study and analysis on overt behavior in order to avoid these problems.

One person who has made many contributions to the study of behavior is B. F. Skinner. Skinner's most important contributions to the science came from his experiments with animals, primarily rats and pigeons, in an experimental chamber sometimes called a Skinner box. This apparatus allowed Skinner to control many, but not all, of the stimuli or activities in the environment and to *observe, measure,* and *experiment with* the responses made by the animal. The use of these controls made it possible to conduct experiments that were similar to the experiments done in physics and chemistry. He and other psychologists developed some very important principles (in the course of experiments) that are discussed in detail in later units.

As an example of experiments conduct by Skinner and the methodology he used, imagine you wanted to know the conditions (experiences) that affect the eating response of a rat. What steps or procedures would be required to produce the answers? First, you'd need to know how much food a rat will eat when both the food and the water are available all the time. You would observe the rat and record the amount of food it eats each day when both food and water are available. This period of observation before any changes are made is called a *baseline*. Next, you would remove the rat's water from its cage and allow it to drink for 15 minutes at 12 noon and 12 midnight. What do you think will happen to the rat's eating response? Will it increase or decrease?

In order to compare the *baseline* (or the amount of food eaten when water was freely available) to the *experimental* condition (when water was available for a limited time), you could construct a *graph*. A graph is a picture that represents the number of responses in each condition. Now, if you actually did the experiment, you should be able to see the effects of depriving the rat of water by looking at the graph. The graph can also be used to tell others the results of the study. After all, what good would it do for a single person or small group of people to know something that may be important to others? In order to inform others of the results, you could describe the experiment (including the graphs), and ask that it be printed in a technical journal. These journal articles contain much important information about the study. Two of the most important pieces of information are (1) the *definition* of the response being studied, and (2) how the response frequency is *measured.*

Response definitions are used to describe the behavior in question. The description includes all the overt characteristics in great detail. This is done so that if two or more people are interested in the same behavior, they can agree as to whether or not it occurs. For example, let's define the eating behavior of the rat. Obviously, the rat must be near enough to the food for it to hold it in its paws and it must be touching the food with its mouth. Does this definition cover all instances of eating behavior? If you were observing a rat's behavior could you use this definition to decide if it was eating?

A *response definition* is a way of specifying what a word (or sometimes a number) means. As we go on in this manual, it will become clear that the meanings of words are just as important to us in our everyday lives as they are to the scientist doing an experiment. We use words to communicate ideas, feelings, wishes, plans, and so on, to our friends, parents, and other people. In doing so, it is important that those words mean basically the same thing to everyone involved; otherwise there could be confusion and arguments about what was really said. Clear response definitions are a way of avoiding such problems in research, and they can be very helpful in our daily lives as well. For example, in the accompanying cartoon from *Tumbleweeds,* the princess probably wishes she had been a little more specific about what she meant when she told Bucolic Buffalo that he lacked tenderness.

You can probably think of times when you said something that was clear to you, but somehow other people misunderstood what you meant. Just because we both use the same word(s), it does not guarantee that we mean the same thing. At this point, we return to the discussion of research techniques, but the importance of clearly specifying what you mean is mentioned again many times in this book.

Once the behavior is defined, it is necessary to find some way to *measure* how often it occurs. There are many ways to do this, but two primary methods are called *frequency* and *duration.* Each method has different rules that define what type of behavior it will accurately measure.

The *frequency method* is best used with responses that are *discrete*; that is, they have a definite beginning and end, and they occur for a relatively constant duration each time. For instance, let's say that you are

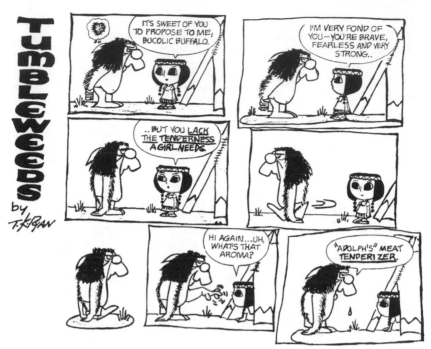

Reprinted with special permission of North American Syndicate.

interested in how many times the phone is used in your home between 7:00 and 8:00 on a Wednesday night. What you would need is a piece of paper divided into two parts on which to keep your data. One part could be labeled "incoming calls" and the other "outgoing calls." Now you should sit somewhere out of the way where you can see and hear the phone. Beginning at 7:00 you should put a mark under incoming phone calls every time the phone rings and a mark under outgoing calls if someone uses the phone to call out. As you collect the data, you will probably notice that the definition does not fit all instances of phone use. You will need to make up *recording rules* for times that do not fit the definition. For example, how will you count a response that consists of (1) picking up the receiver and replacing it without dialing; or (2) if the phone rings, and no one is on the other end; finally, (3) if the phone rings, and the caller has the wrong number? The rule could be as follows: For outgoing calls, the caller must dial all seven numbers, and incoming calls need to be answered with the caller still on the line.

The second method used to measure behavior is called the *duration method*. It is different from frequency because it is used for *continuous* responses—responses that continue or last over long periods of time. An example of a response for which you would use the duration method is how much time a person spends working on his/her homework. First you need to define the homework behavior. Probably you would want to include a setting (i.e., where the studying will take place), the materials needed (e.g., books, paper, and something with which to write). You would need a watch to time the behavior from whenever the person who is to study sits down and either opens a book or begins to write. When the individual stops and gets up, the time is then stopped and recorded on a piece of paper. Can you think of some recording rules you would need to make? How about if the person remains in the chair and begins to stare at the ceiling—is this studying? It will depend on how you wish to define studying.

There are, then, two major differences between these methods. The *frequency* method is based on discrete responses while the *duration* method is based on continuous responses. The frequency method is used to see how *often* a response occurs. The duration method is used if you are interested in how *long* a response lasts.

Now that the two basic methods of recording data have been specified, can you think of some reasons why measurement is important? Consider the example of the number of phone calls. Suppose that there is a conflict between the parents and a teenager in the family over the phone. The parents state that the teenager is on the phone too many times during the evening. The teenager disagrees; so the parents and teenager agree to collect some data in order to deal with the problem fairly. If you were the teenager, which method would you use to collect data? Because the problem is too many calls and not necessarily the length of calls, you would want to use the frequency method. The data collected are called a *baseline* because you haven't done anything to the occurrence of phone calls. Once the data are collected, there is an objective basis for deciding whether there actually is a problem or not. The teenager may be using the phone too much, or on the other hand, the parents could have been mistaken. Rather than fighting about the phone, the data can be used to decide how many phone calls are too many. Perhaps everyone would agree that the teenager could make or receive a total of two phone calls an evening (after 6:00 P.M.), but any calls over two would cost $.50 each. The family would then collect data on the teenager's phone calls again to see if this change (the experimental condition) had any effect on the number of calls made each night.

There is one other method of collecting information about a response or behavior that does not involve directly observing the behavior. This method is called *outcome measurement*. The behavior produces a

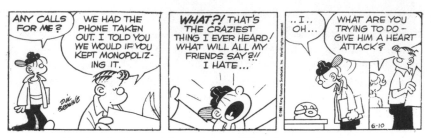

Reprinted with special permission of King Features Syndicate.

product or change that can later be measured. For example, in the case of the rat's eating response, we could simply weigh the amount of food we give it in the morning and weigh the food again in the evening. The difference in the weight would tell us how much food the rat ate. Of course it is not quite as simple as that; we would have to make sure that the rate was not dropping the food or hiding it in the nest. It is important to note that this method does not provide information on how many times the rat ate or how long it spent eating the food; but if knowing how much was eaten was all that was important, it could be measured this way.

Outcome measurement can be very useful and can save a lot of time. For example, if your class was concerned about littering in the school cafeteria during lunch periods, there are several ways to collect the data. The class could try to count each time someone dropped a piece of trash, but it probably would be easier and more reliable to simply count the number of pieces of trash in the cafeteria before and after the lunch period. This information could then be used to decide whether the cafeteria was getting cleaner or messier.

The major reason for defining and measuring events is so that there will be an objective basis for deciding what is happening.

Study Guide

Use these words to fill in the blanks (each word may be used more than once or not at all):

a. baseline	e. behavior	i. continuous	m. define
b. measure	f. frequency	j. overt	n. discrete
c. duration	g. graph	k. covert	
d. science	h. observe	l. experiment	

1. Psychology is a _____ that

   studies _____.

2. Behavior we can see is called _____;
   behavior we cannot see is called

   _____.
   Walking is an observable behavior so we say it is an

   _____ behavior. Singing, crying,

   and playing tennis are _____ be-
   haviors. Thinking cannot be observed. Thinking is an example of a

   _____ behavior.
3. The experimental chamber controls for activities in the environment

   so that psychologists can _____,

   _____, and

   _____ with behavior.

4. The record of a behavior before an experimental condition is called a

   _____.

5. A _____ is a picture that repre-
   sents a number form of the amount of response in a condition.

6. A response definition is used to

   _____ a behavior.

7. The frequency method is best used with responses that are

   _____.

8. When you are interested in the length of time a response lasts, you

   should use the _____ method.

9. The duration method is used for responses that are

   _____.

10. Bill's best friend, John, seemed to be girl crazy. Bill got tired of
    hearing about girls all the time and wanted John to realize how much

he talked about them. Bill decided to count the number of times John spoke about girls and the number of times he spoke about other subjects. Is this method of measuring behavior the frequency or the duration method? _____

11. If Bill kept track of the length of time John spoke about girls, he would be using the _____ method.

12. Jill wanted to count the number of times she said something nice to another person during the day. This would be an example of the _____ method.

13. Rosemary was overweight. She wanted to find out how many minutes each day she spends eating. What method of measuring would she be using? _____

14. Gary thinks his father watches TV too much. Gary would like his father to spend more time shooting baskets or playing catch with him. Gary decides to keep a record of the time his father spends watching TV each week. What method would this be?

_____

15. When Bill kept track of the number of times John spoke about girls, he was actually recording the

_____. (This is the period of observation before any changes are made.)

UNIT 2

Measurement and Definition of Behavior Exercise

Ruby was 10 years old. She had a little brother who was 6. Ruby frequently hit him and made him cry. Her mother and father became concerned and decided to do something about her behavior. So they consulted a psychologist who, along with many other things, told them to count the number of times they actually saw Ruby hit her brother. The first thing the parents and the psychologist had to do was define hitting behavior. (As part of your assignment, try to write a behavioral definition of hitting. Be sure and decide what kinds of behaviors should be included under hitting. For example, if Ruby uses her elbows to strike her brother, is that a hit? How hard does a blow have to be before it is a hit?) They counted the occurrence of hitting for 5 days, and the data (number of hits each day) were as follows: 25, 20, 29, 34, 32. They then went back to the psychologist with the data. The psychologist suggested the parents try to be nice to Ruby when she was not hitting her brother and also to use a procedure called time-out to see if this could decrease the amount of hitting, and collect data for five more days. In the time-out procedure, each time she hit her brother, Ruby had to sit in a chair at the dining room table and do nothing at all. She also had to go to bed 5 minutes early for each hit.

The data for the next 5 days looked like this: 15, 7, 3, 5, 2. They then returned to the psychologist with the data. The psychologist said that it looked like the time-out and the reinforcement of appropriate behavior were working, but to make sure, it was suggested that they stop the procedures to see what would happen to Ruby's frequency of hitting. When they stopped the procedures, Ruby's frequency of hitting again

increased. The data for the period were as follows: 10, 8, 13, 37, 40, 30.
The psychologist quickly suggested they go back to using time-out and
reinforcing Ruby when she was nice, and within 5 days, Ruby stopped
hitting her brother. The data for those days, were 10, 7, 3, 0, and 0 hits.

　　A graph representing the results of this study has been started at the
bottom of this page. The axes have been labeled "Number of Hits per
Day" (ordinate axis) and "Days" (abscissa) and the data for the first
baseline have been placed. Finish the graph by labeling the remaining
conditions, "Treatment 1," "Baseline 2," and "Treatment 2" and then
putting the rest of the data points on the figure. After you have finished
the graph, decide whether the procedures suggested by the psychologist
had any effect on Ruby's hitting behavior. Use the graph form provided

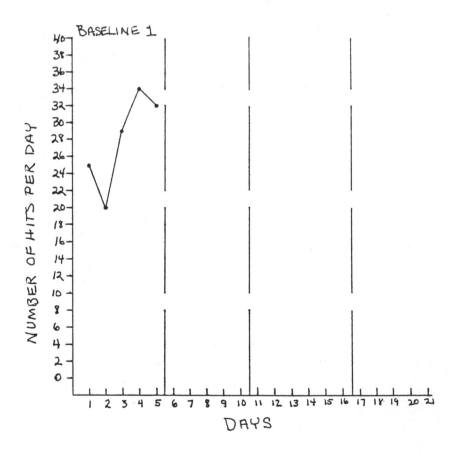

for you, and write your own behavioral definition of hitting and your evaluation of whether the procedures were helping Ruby, on the back.

The preceding example was simplified for this exercise. The psychologist and the parents did many other things to help Ruby, but the first step was to reduce the number of times she hit her brother.

UNIT 3

The Experimental Method

The experiment is the key element of science. In fact, science and our modern society could never have evolved as they have without the development of the experiment. The experiment allows the scientist to manipulate variables and to draw inferences about the causes of particular events. Before scientists began using the experimental method, arguments over the causes of phenomena were usually decided by who was the most persuasive speaker or writer (or perhaps the loudest or biggest).

For example, during the time of Galileo, the great Renaissance scientist, it was standard practice for people of learning to base all of their arguments on the writing of Aristotle. Aristotle was the greatest of the early Greek philosophers and perfected the form of deductive logic called the syllogism. Aristotle also wrote extensively on almost every topic, and although he was often correct in his logical deductions, he was more often wrong. Because just about all of the early Renaissance philosophers simply accepted all of Aristotle's arguments as true, they were unable to tell when he was right or wrong.

Galileo, however, was more interested in actually testing explanations to see if they worked, regardless of whether they agreed with Aristotle. One famous incident between Galileo and his colleagues concerned Aristotle's prediction that a 10-pound weight should fall 10 times faster than a 1-pound weight.[2] One day Galileo climbed to the top of the Tower of Pisa, and as his adversaries were walking by he yelled and dropped a 10-pound and 1-pound weight at the same time. The two weights hit the ground almost simultaneously, thus experimentally dis-

2. Some science historians have suggested that this incident never actually took place. However, because the story clearly illustrates testing versus simply accepting an explanation, it is presented as an example, whether or not it is true.

proving Aristotle's prediction. Interestingly enough, the other professors were so committed to their belief in Aristotle that they decided their eyes must have deceived them rather than accepting that Aristotle had been wrong. Unfortunately, even today, scientific evidence is rejected when that evidence contradicts strongly held beliefs.

The experiment has become more complex since Galileo's early efforts. One of the individuals most responsible for the development of the experimental method was the great French scientist, Louis Pasteur. Pasteur was trained as a physical chemist, but his interests gradually shifted to problems of biology and medicine. Although he was not a physician, Pasteur had a profound effect on medicine, in that he developed the microorganism theory of disease. Through his research and that of others, it was possible to identify the various bacteria and microbes responsible for such diseases as cholera, tuberculosis, diphtheria, pneumonia, and scarlet fever. The discovery of these microorganisms led to a revolution in the treatment of disease and health care in general. Pasteur also furthered the development of preventive medicine by pioneering research on inoculation. Specifically, he produced a vaccine to make a person immune to rabies (hydrophobia), a terrible disease that causes the victim to die in agony. The story of Pasteur's life and his accomplishments make exciting and fascinating reading. If you are interested in the development of the rabies vaccine or Pasteur's research on microbes, you should ask the school librarian for a copy of one of the fine books on Pasteur.

Pasteur's experimental method can be seen in how he studied the problem of spoiling wine. The wine industry is very important in France. And in the 19th century, the French Navy tried to keep their sailors happy by providing them with a daily ration of wine. Unfortunately for the Navy, the wine was all spoiling, which of course didn't make the sailors very happy. So with both unhappy wine producers and unhappy sailors, the French government asked Pasteur to investigate the problem. He first compared the spoiled wine to the good wine and found that the spoiled wine was cloudy and had particles suspended in it. Pasteur suspected that some type of bacteria was causing the wine to spoil, so he placed a small amount of bad wine in some good wine. The particles of the bad wine quickly multiplied in the new wine and soon it was spoiled as well. Next, he took some bad wine and boiled it (sterilizing the wine). He reasoned that if the spoilage was caused by bacteria, heating the wine would kill them. He then placed a drop of the boiled (sterilized) wine in some good wine and it did not spoil! The results of these experiments seemed to support his interpretation that bacteria was causing the wine to spoil, so he asked the Navy to conduct an applied experiment. The Navy took a batch of new wine and boiled half of it. The wine was then placed on a ship for a long voyage. The wine was checked when the ship returned and the boiled wine stayed fine while the other wine had spoiled. Pasteur's hypothesis about microorganisms causing the spoilage was verified. The French wine industry introduced sterilization into their procedures and once again the French sailors were happy.

For many years, psychologists did not use experiments to analyze human behavior—one wouldn't like a psychologist to boil or drop children from great heights to see how the experience affected them. Seriously, there are important moral and ethical issues that must be considered when experiments are conducted using humans as the subjects. Great care must be taken so that the individual benefits from participating in the research and that he/she is not unduly exposed to experiences that are likely to cause physical or psychological harm.

One experiment that illustrates psychological research is the "Case of Cathy the Crawler." Cathy was an attractive little girl who attended a preschool run by a university institute of child development. The institute studied the way the children act at various ages and in particular situations. Cathy was attending this preschool because of some unusual behaviors or responses she consistently displayed. Cathy spent almost all of her time crawling around both inside and outside the preschool. She very seldom got up and ran around with the other kids, even though she could walk and run just as well as any of them. If Cathy had been 1 or 2 years old, probably no one would have worried about her crawling, but Cathy was 4½ and she had been crawling around like this for about a year.

The preschool teachers thought that Cathy's crawling was a symptom of psychological disturbance. Specifically, crawling was a sign of Cathy's regression to an earlier stage of development (infancy) because she was unhappy. When someone is unhappy, you try to make them happy. So when Cathy would crawl, the teachers would attend to her, try to encourage her, in short, try to make her happy. On the other hand, the psychologists thought Cathy might be crawling *because* the teachers attended to her when she was crawling and not at other times. How could you design an experiment to see if attention was causing Cathy to crawl? Well, the psychologists decided simply to change the behavior that would produce teacher attention for Cathy. From now on, the teachers were only to attend to Cathy when she was standing and ignore her when she was crawling. After a few days of this, Cathy was standing most of the time and only occasionally crawling. Soon Cathy was playing like all of the other children. The full experiment was more complex than this, but in summary, by changing what behavior produced the attention, the psychologists were able to prove that it was the attention that was causing Cathy to crawl and not some psychological disorder.

The essence of the experiment is having an idea and testing it in someway. That is, the experimenter first identifies some event or process (a variable such as introducing bacteria into wine) that may be responsible for (cause) the occurrence of some other event (e.g., bacteria causes wine to spoil). Next, the variable is changed (manipulated in some way) to see how that manipulation affects the occurrence of the second event.

The experiment may be as simple as Galileo's dropping the two weights. Here, Aristotle argued that weight would affect how fast an object fell in direct proportion to its weight. Galileo simply took two weights and dropped them to see if it was true. If the heavier one had fallen much faster than the other, Aristotle would have been correct. But because they fell at almost exactly the same rate, he was proven wrong.

Similarly, Pasteur hypothesized that it was bacteria causing the wine to spoil. One way of testing this idea was to kill the bacteria in some wine by heating it and to leave the bacteria in other wine alone. The treated wine did not spoil, while the untreated wine did. No need for arguments here. The results are quite clear, and a new treatment for keeping liquids from spoiling (pasteurization) was developed.

Finally, another form of experiment was demonstrated by the psychologists working with Cathy. They systematically changed which of Cathy's behaviors could attract the teachers' attention. When Cathy's behavior changed, it proved that it was the teachers' attention that was responsible for the way Cathy acted and not some other variable.

Over the course of this program, you will have the opportunity to do simple experiments. In those experiments, you will be trying to analyze some psychological phenomena. The first step is to identify some variable or event you think may be important in the problem. Next, you manipulate that variable in some way. Finally, you observe to see if the manipulation produces the effects you expected. If it does, then your analysis of the problem was correct. If it doesn't work out as you expected, you learned something new about the problem. If the first thing you try doesn't work, rethink the problem and try again by changing something new. Remember that no experiment is ever really a failure because it also helps to know what doesn't work.

In looking at the lives of great scientists, it becomes clear that the second most important characteristic they all share is persistence (after intelligence). So when you start your experiment, *don't* give up if it doesn't work the first time—keep trying.

Study Guide

1. A key element of science is the

   _____.

2. Experiments are conducted to test

   _____.

3. Galileo conducted a simple experiment to test Aristotle's explanation
   of how objects of different _____
   will fall.

4. He dropped two objects of different weights and they landed at the
   _____ time.

5. This result _____ Aristotle's explanation.

6. Pasteur was a great scientist who developed the
   _____ theory of disease.

7. He conducted some interesting experiments on why wine

   _____.

8. In the wine experiments, Pasteur
   _____ the important variable by
   boiling one batch of wine and not the other.

9. Cathy was a little girl of 4½ who spent most of her time

   _____.

10. The teachers thought Cathy crawled because she was unhappy so they
    _____ to her when she crawled.

11. The psychologists thought Cathy crawled because the teacher
    _____ to her crawling.

12. To test their idea, the psychologists had the teachers attend to Cathy only when she was _____.

13. The results of the experiment demonstrated that Cathy crawled because teachers' _____ was delivered when she crawled.

14. List the three major steps of an experiment.

   a. _____

   b. _____

   c. _____

A Psychological Experiment in Social Interaction

The following pages give detailed instructions on how to conduct and analyze a simple psychological experiment. The experiment you are about to conduct is a version of a very important study done by a psychologist, Dr. Joel Greenspoon, in 1956. Because the results of psychological experiments can be biased by the experimenter's expectations, we will not tell you anything about Greenspoon's results. For the experiment, you will need three people: the experimenter, an observer, and someone to be the subject. If you are selected to be the subject, you will not be given any detailed information about how the experiment will work. Basically, the subject will be asked to leave the room for a while so that the experimenter and the observer can get ready. You will then be asked to come back and talk to the experimenter about everything you did last week. The experiment is about how certain psychological procedures affect conversations. Sometimes the experimenter may say something to you and other times he/she may just listen. However, you will not be asked to do anything that will embarrass you, nor will you be tricked in any way. But remember, your cooperation is necessary for the experiment to work.

Subjects should not read any further at this time.

Instructions for the Experimenter and Observer

This is a study of the effects of verbal consequences—such as "mmhum," "that's interesting," "uhuh," and "how nice"— on the verbal responses of another person. When we speak to people, we often use these phrases. Greenspoon was interested in how these responses would affect the person you talk to. Greenspoon picked out a particular class of verbal responses such as plural nouns or color names and every time the person he was talking to said one of those words he said mmhum and how interesting, etc. For your experiment we will use plural nouns as the response class. Plural nouns are words such as cars, boats, sisters, shoes, dishes, geese, men, and women.

Specific Instructions for the Observers

You will need a piece of paper with 15 lines on it, one for each minute of the experiment, a watch, and a pencil. When the experiment starts, you will record with a tally mark (/) each time the subject says a plural noun. You will record each minute separately, so you will need to watch the time while you are listening and move to the next line at the end of each minute. **Do not read the experimenter's instructions.**

Specific Instructions for the Experimenter

The experimenter will need a table, two chairs, and a watch. Bring the subject back into the room, have the subject sit on the other side of the table, and ask him/her to relax. Explain that you want him/her to tell you everything he/she did last week. Explain that the experiment will last 15 minutes and that during that time you will listen and occasionally comment. Ask if there are any questions, then tell the subject to start. For the first *5 minutes*, you will just listen in a positive but noncommittal manner. After 5 minutes *have passed* (use your watch to time the experiment, but don't let the subject see you doing it) *each time* the subject says a *plural noun*, you are to immediately say "mmhum," "uhuh," "how interesting," "that's interesting," "how nice." In other words, you should show interest every time the person says a plural noun, but at all other times you will just listen and not say anything. You will use this procedure for 5 minutes and then stop. For the last 5 minutes, you again will *only* listen. After 15 minutes, tell the subject that the experiment is over.

Now all of you (the subject, the observer, and the experimenter) can look at and analyze the data. The data are the number of times the subject said a plural noun in each minute. For the analysis, you will need a sheet of graph paper. Label the vertical axis (the ordinate) "Number of Plural Nouns" and use two squares to represent each plural noun. Label the horizontal axis (the abscissa) "Minutes." There will be 15 spaces here, 1 for each minute of the experiment. Your graph should now look like the graph at the top of page 25.

Next, draw a vertical line between Minutes 5 and 6 and another one between Minutes 10 and 11. These lines will show when the experimenter was commenting after each plural noun. Now take the data from the record sheet and put those data on the graph. An example data sheet and graph are at the bottom of page 25.

Your data should look something like the hypothetical data presented here. What do you think they mean? Greenspoon discovered that each time he made comments showing interest after learning a plural noun, the subject said more plural nouns; when he stopped, the subject stopped also. Analyze your own results and see if they are similar. Then write out three ideas that you think might explain why this happened. We discuss the results of Greenspoon's study in the unit on positive and negative reinforcement (Unit 7).

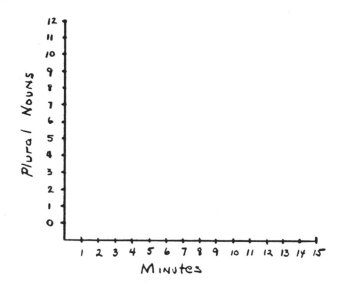

Minutes

Data Sheet

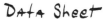

1. —	6. /	11. ⫽⫽⫽ /
2. /	7. ///	12. ///
3. //	8. ⫽⫽⫽ ////	13. ////
4. /	9. ⫽⫽⫽ //	14. /
5. —	10. ⫽⫽⫽ ////	15. —

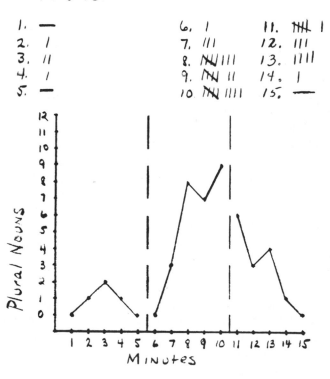

Minutes

UNIT 5

Understanding Causes: The Relevance of the Experimental Method to Everyday Life

We have just examined some ways the experimental method is used in science to develop explanations of why an event occurred. Put another way, the experiment is used to discover causes of phenomena. Concern about causes, however, is not limited to scientists; many times a day, we each ask why this or that happened. You may not have thought about it in this fashion, but the questions, "Why do I have a headache?" "Why doesn't the TV work?" and "Why is Susan so unfriendly?" are all really questions about the causes of those events.

The answers we accept for such questions depends on how important the particular question is to us and our knowledge of the topic. Susan's unfriendly behavior may produce mild curiosity if we only meet her casually, but it will be of great concern if she is our sister. In the casual situation, being told that Susan is a hostile person will satisfy our curiosity and suggest that she should be avoided in the future. On the other hand, such an explanation will be of little help to Susan's sisters and brothers. They will need to know many more specific reasons (causes) for her unfriendly behavior if they hope to be happy living with her.

How do we go about discovering answers to our questions about causes? There appear to be three main sources or types of explanations used in everyday life: (1) *authority/common sense*, (2) *contiguity and correlation*, and (3) *experimental/logical analysis*. Although they are often used in combination, we examined them separately here to clarify the differences among them.

Authority and common sense are paired here not because the two forms of explanation are developed in exactly the same way but because we accept and use them for similar reasons. Explanations via authority or common sense are given to us by other people; we do not produce them for ourselves. First, we have a question about why something, Y, is happening or has happened, and then we are told X is the reason why Y is occurring or has occurred. We are told that Sally gets good grades because she is smart (common sense) or that the Son of Sam killed because he is a paranoid schizophrenic (authority in the form of psychiatric testimony). These assertions seem to make sense and, therefore, are accepted as the explanation for the events in question. Two factors are important in determining whether we accept such explanations. First, is the explanation consistent (does it fit) with other things we believe? And second, does the explanation come from someone we recognize as an authority? Obviously, it does not have to come from a Nobel prize winner; parents, teachers, older siblings, peers, and a variety of other persons often function as authorities in everyday life. Thus, if the explanation both comes from someone whom we respect and makes sense, we are likely to accept it.

You should have noticed, however, that neither of these criteria have anything to do with whether the explanation is correct. Remember the idea that a 10-pound weight would fall 10 times faster than a 1-pound weight was generally accepted because Aristotle had said so and because it made sense to the scholars of the time. The tendency to accept authoritative or common sense answers can sometimes produce tragic results. For instance, as late as the 17th century, it was both authoritatively correct and commonly held that witches were the cause of unusual illness or strange behavior. When someone suddenly became sick for no apparent reason, it was often assumed by both the formal authorities (government and church) and the community as a whole that witchcraft was the cause. This explanation had two very undesirable consequences. Most obviously, many innocent people were executed as witches. Further, a less obvious but probably more important result was that as long as witchcraft was accepted as the cause of unusual illnesses, no other causes were sought or treatments developed. Thus, many people whose illnesses might have been cured died because the focus of treatment was on finding the witch and not on treating the illness per se. Although from our perspective believing in witchcraft may seem foolish, it is undoubtedly the case that at some future date, our descendants will look back at some of our currently held beliefs and explanations and wonder, "How could anyone be so stupid?"

Although an uncritical reliance on authority often leads to problems, authoritative explanations can nevertheless be a source of much useful information. This is especially the case when common sense and authority are used in the more systematic fashion called *deduction*. Returning to the question of why the television set doesn't work, an instruction book probably came with the set. The instruction book is a form of authoritative information, in that it tells us possible reasons why the television is not working and how to fix it. We can, therefore, check it for both an explanation and ways of getting the television to work. From the description in the book, we get an idea or hypothesis about why the set is not working and then check it by trying it out. If this fixes the set, fine. If not, we may try something else suggested by the manual or take the set to the repair shop to be fixed. The technician will then use essentially the same procedures, but the process will be based on the much more technically detailed manuals that he/she has been specifically trained to use.

Interestingly enough, in modern medicine, the doctor will go about treating illnesses in a very similar fashion, using tests to identify the problem and then treating it in the method suggested by the texts. The major difference between these uses of authority and the simple acceptance of authoritative or common sense explanations is that the technician and the physician systematically test to see whether the explanation is correct in terms of fixing the set or curing the illness.

A second common source of explanations is the contiguity of two events in time. *Contiguity* means that two events are observed to occur together, usually with one slightly preceding the other. We observe a baseball hit a window and the window breaking. The obvious—and in this case correct—interpretation of the events is that the ball making contact with the window at a particular force caused the window to break. The closely timed linkage of events leads us to conclude that the first event is the cause of the second.

An even more striking example of such causal interpretation involves the contiguity between eating novel foods and illness. Suppose you have never eaten oysters before, but a friend convinces you to try them. After eating a batch of oysters, you become very sick and spend the rest of the day throwing up. You conclude that the oysters made you sick. Are you correct in this conclusion? Possibly—it could very well be that you are allergic to oysters or that this was a bad batch. Alternatively, it may have been something else that you ate with the oysters that made you sick. Further, the cause of your illness may have been totally independent of your eating—for example, the beginning of the flu. The reason we almost always decide that it was the oysters is because of the easily observed contiguity between eating the oysters and becoming sick.

The example of the oysters illustrates both the strength of our tendency to interpret contiguity as cause, and the possibly misleading consequences of that interpretation. The problem with using contiguity as the basis for judging causes is that the sequence of the two events could have occurred by accident. Suppose you observe your brother talking to your mother and then she immediately calls you and bawls you out for something. What are you likely to conclude is the reason for your being bawled out? It is a safe bet that later in the day, you and your brother will have a fight over the injustice he has done you. But what if your mother was already on her way to punish you and your brother just happened to stop to talk about something totally unrelated to you? Or perhaps he saw she was really mad at you and stopped her to try to intervene on your behalf. (You may judge this to be very unlikely, but stranger things have happened.) If either of these is the reason for your brother talking to your mother, then you and he will get into a needless fight.

Although the contiguity between two interesting events should not automatically be interpreted in terms of X causing Y, it does give you a place to start your search for a cause or causes. Instead of relying on just the one observation of the two events occurring together, we could try to make many observations of both X and Y. Do X and Y always occur together? Does Y sometimes occur without X? Does X occur without being followed by Y? When we carefully observe two events in order to answer these questions, we are doing a correlational analysis. A *correlation* is a measure of the relation or interdependency of two events. A correlation of 1.0 would mean that every time X occurs, Y follows; whereas a 0 correlation means that Y *never* follows X. Absolute correlations of 1 or 0 are very rare, and the correlations between most events are low. Therefore, even a correlation (r) of 0.3 is usually large enough for a scientist to conclude that the two events are related in some fashion. So if we were to observe systematically the occurrences of your brother speaking to your mother and also your mother punishing you, and found a correlation of $r = 0.5$, then we would be fairly confident that there is some relation between your brother's behavior and your punishment.

Notice that it was not concluded that your brother was causing your mother to punish you, only that the two events were *probably* related. For any correlation, there are at least four possible explanations. The first is the spurious or accidental correlation where the two events were not really related but only appear to be mathematically. A famous example of a spurious correlation was the very high correlation found for the years 1950–1960 between the number of rabbits in Australia and the Dow Jones stock price index. It is very difficult to imagine how increases or decreases in the rabbit population could cause the prices of stocks to similarly increase or decrease. In the same manner, the correlation between your mother talking to your brother before punishing you may be accidental (spurious). Perhaps he spends most of his time in a room she has to pass through to come talk to you. Her talking to him first, then, is a result of the physical arrangement of the house and not the cause of your being punished.

On the other hand, your worst suspicions may be correct: He is in fact saying things to your mother that sometimes causes her to punish you. This is the standard interpretation of a correlation: Event X (brother talking to mother) apparently occurring before event Y (punishment) is taken to be the cause of Y. But what if Y were the cause of X? Your mother on her way to punish you (i.e., the decision has already been made) stops to warn your brother not to do such a thing himself or he too will be punished. In other words, your punishment is really the cause of her stopping to talk to your brother. Finally, some other factor, Z, may be causing both your punishment and the conversation with your brother. Perhaps it is your father who decides when you should be punished and your brother warned. If that is correct, then X and Y are not causally related at all; father Z is the cause of both X and Y. As a consequence, it is important to remember that the observation of two events occurring together does not necessarily mean that one is the cause of the other.

Based on the observed correlation between X and Y, four possible interpretations exist.

1. X and Y are not really related; the correlation is spurious or accidental.
2. X is a cause of Y.
3. Y is a cause of X.
4. Some other factor, Z, is the cause of both X and Y.

If we wish to be certain about why a particular event occurs, then the most effective way of determining its causes is the experiment. Experiments can be very complex or simple depending on the nature of the questions and how certain we must be about the answers. The experiments being conducted in physics to discover the nature of subatomic particles and the forces that hold them together can cost millions of dollars. On the other hand, many of my experiments just cost a small amount for materials and the volunteer time of individuals such as yourselves. Nonetheless, the principles are the same; we each try to manipulate the variable thought to be causing the events in question. For example, if we wished to know if the oysters had caused you to become ill, the experiment to answer that question would manipulate the presence or absence of oysters in your diet. This could be done in several ways. In the simplest, we could grind them up and fry them in a batter to disguise the physical characteristics without changing their biochemical features. Then, on a random schedule of days, we would give you fritters that contain oysters or ones without oysters. If you became ill on days when the oysters were present and not when they were absent, we would know that something in oysters makes you sick. Similarly, if you never got sick, then it was something other than oysters that made you sick the first time. There are many experiments that could be done to explore the characteristics of oysters as food, but all of them would involve some similar manipulation of an aspect of the oyster (e.g., visual characteristics or how they smell).

If you really wanted to find out if your brother was influencing your mother, you could send him off somewhere for a couple of weeks to see if the frequency of punishment decreased. Again, however, other factors could affect the results (e.g., the amount of work your parents must do to care for one less child; the amount of time available for paying attention to your behaviors that may be punishable), but that experiment will be left for later. Because much of the rest of the book is designed to teach you how you can use simple experiments to solve everyday problems, further details about the experimental method are not presented here. The main point is that every day we have questions about and develop explanations for the things that happen to us. The more we understand about how scientific decisions are made, the better we are able to understand and control our own lives.

Shoe ━━━━

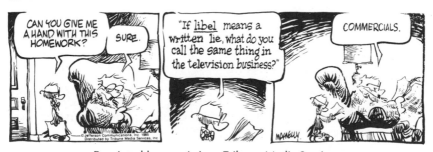

Reprinted by permission: Tribune Media Services.

Study Guide

1. Questions of why are really about the

   _____ of those events.

2. What are explanations given to us by other people called?

   _____

3. What are the reasons we accept authoritative explanations?

   _____

4. _____ is when two events occur
   together in time.

5. When events are contiguous, the first is often taken as the
   _____ of the second.

6. The occurrence of two events together may have been the result of

   _____.

7. A correlation is a measure of how

   _____ two events are.

8. List the *four* possible explanations of a correlation.

   a. _____

   b. _____

   c. _____

   d. _____

9. If you wish to be certain of why something occurs, you should
   conduct an _____.

10. In an experiment, the hypothesized cause is

    _____ to determine its effect on the
    phenomenon.

11. What are some reasons for being skeptical about authoritative or com-
    mon sense explanations? _____

    _____

UNIT 6

Operant Behavior and Consequences

Thus far, we have discussed the importance of the procedures involved in defining, measuring, and manipulating variables for the development of science in general. We now begin to examine systematically the role these procedures play in the science of psychology, and how psychology is relevant to your everyday life. Psychology is a very broad field covering many phenomena such as the effects of neural transmitters on behavior, the psychophysics of hearing, or the hallucinations of paranoid schizophrenics. Although these and other phenomena are very important, they probably do not have much direct relevance to you on a daily basis. As a consequence, we focus our coverage of psychology on what is called operant behavior.

Some examples of operant behavior are smiling, running, reading, dressing, driving a car, and so on. Operant behavior sometimes is called voluntary behavior. There are two basic reasons for calling these responses voluntary. First, we know they are not reflexes or instincts, which are involuntary. Instincts and reflexes are responses that are not learned as the person grows up but rather are determined by genetic (inherited) factors. An example of a reflex is the pupil's response to a bright light. If you shine a light into a person's eye, the pupil will contract (get smaller). You don't have to learn this response; it seems to be built in. Also, unless there is something wrong with the person (e.g., a brain concussion), the response will occur every time you shine a light into the eye. Instincts are similar to reflexes but usually a little more complex.

It is easy to see, however, that operant responses such as smiling are not involuntary reflexes or instincts. The easiest test to determine whether a response is a reflex or an instinct is to ask, "Is there a single stimulus that always produces this particular response?" For the pupillary reflex, the answer is yes, but for a smile, the answer is clearly no. Second, we often explain these behaviors in terms of our wishes (e.g., "I did it because I wanted to"), or we make statements concerning our intention to engage in some activity (e.g., "I am going swimming"). These terms imply what can be called *voluntary* control. Although, as scientists, we do not know how important our wishes or desires are in determining how we act, we do know the consequences that follow operant behaviors are very important in determining whether we engage in those behaviors again in the future.

In the case of smiling, suppose I smile at someone and that person smiles back and says, "Hello, how are you?" in a very pleasant manner as we pass. In the future, I am likely to smile at that person again. If, however, the individual says in a very unpleasant way, "What are you smiling at?" Are you some kind of wise guy?" I am probably not going to smile at that person again. Similarly, if I go to a party with some new acquaintances and have a terrible time, I probably won't go to the same type of party again in the near future. If, on the other hand, I have a terrific time, I will probably start looking for a new party the next day. It should be clear from these examples that the term *consequences* simply means what happens after I do something. In discussing operant behavior, we divide consequences into three categories: positive reinforcers,

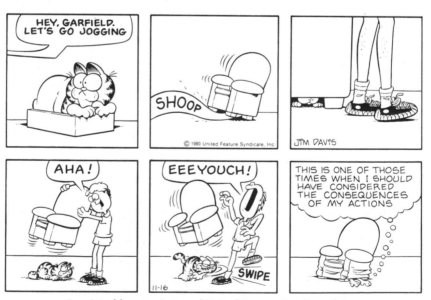

Reprinted by permission of United Feature Syndicated, Inc.

negative reinforcers, and neutral stimuli. How these consequences can be manipulated to affect operant behaviors is discussed in the next few units. In the mean time, we thought you might enjoy the accompanying cartoon, which illustrates how Garfield discovered that consequences are very important.

Study Guide

1. Instincts and reflexes are called

   _____ responses.

2. Basic instincts and reflexes appear to be inherited or

   _____.

3. Operant behavior is called

   _____.

4. Operant responses are affected by

   _____.

5. Consequences are stimuli that

   _____ a response.

6. What were the consequences of Garfield's actions?

   _____.

UNIT 7

Reinforcement: Positive and Negative

Reinforcement is the process of increasing the frequency of a behavior by changing the consequences that follow the behavior in question. There are two types of reinforcement—positive and negative—but *reinforcement* always results in an *increase* in the frequency of the response that produces the reinforcement.

Earlier, we discussed the experiment with Cathy the Crawler. The psychologists discovered that when the teachers attended to Cathy's crawling, she crawled a lot. But when they ignored her crawling and attended to her when she was standing, she stood most of the time. The results of the experiment indicate that for Cathy, the teacher attention was a *positive reinforcer*. The behavior that produced teacher attention increased in frequency. The process of delivering a positive reinforcer contingent on (i.e., *only* given at that time, but *always* given at that time) the occurrence of a response is called *positive reinforcement*.

This definition sounds very complex, but positive reinforcement is really pretty simple. Although the ideas of reward and reinforcement have been around for a long time, the first psychologist to do systematic research on the process now called positive reinforcement was B. F. Skinner. In a book called *The Behavior of Organisms*, he describes a series of experiments he conducted with rats. The basic experiment was to put a food-deprived (hungry) rat into an experimental chamber that contained a bar and a food container on one wall. The rat would wander around the chamber sniffing, biting, and pushing things as rats commonly do. If the rat happened to push the bar down, food was immediately dropped into the food container. Because the rat was food-deprived, of course the rat ate it and then pressed the bar again. This bar press was also immediately followed by the delivery of food. Soon, the rat was steadily pressing the bar and eating the food. In this case, the food was the *positive reinforcer* and the rat was *deprived* of food except when it pressed the bar. In other words, unless the rat pressed the bar, it didn't get any food. The relationship between the bar press and the delivery of food is called the *contingency*. That is, the food was delivered *every* time the bar was pressed and *only* when the bar was pressed. Under these circumstances, the bar press increased in frequency. The process is called *positive reinforcement*. The rat presses the bar because it produced food in the past. If the bar press is no longer followed by food, after a short period of time, the rat stops pressing the bar. Also, the food (positive reinforcer) must be delivered immediately after the occurrence of the bar press for it to have any effect on the rat's frequency of bar pressing. If we wait a minute after the bar press before delivering the food, the rat probably will not learn to bar press. It might do whatever it was doing immediately before the food was delivered, such as standing on its hind legs in the corner of the chamber. This would happen because standing in the corner was the response that was positively reinforced. In short, if you wish to reinforce a particular behavior, the positive reinforcer must be delivered *immediately* after that response occurs.

In reading about Skinner's experiment with the rat, you should have recognized some similarities between it and the Greenspoon experiment you conducted. In fact, Greenspoon's study was what is called a systematic replication of Skinner's experiment. Instead of rats, Greenspoon worked with people as his subjects. Also, he did not use food as the positive reinforcer, he used what are called *social reinforcers* (i.e., attention, "mmhum," "how nice," etc.). Greenspoon found that when he delivered social attention contingent on the occurrence of plural nouns, the person he was talking to said more plural nouns. Similarly, when he stopped giving social attention, the person slowly stopped saying plural nouns. If your experiment produced similar results then you demonstrated that for your subject, words like "mmhum" or "uhuh," were positive reinforcers that increased the probability of saying plural nouns. (Because you cannot always control every important factor in the experiment, you might not have gotten those results.) The study also shows that how people react to what we say influences what we say to them in the future. When you finish this unit, review the ideas you wrote to explain the results of your experiment, and see if you can now write a better explanation of what happened.

Another illustration of the use of positive reinforcement concerns Danny and his mother. Young Danny was a real slob when it came to leaving his things all over the house. His mother constantly had to nag, yell, and threaten him to keep the house from looking like a garbage dump. In short, Dan was the living personification of the "Pig Pen" character in the *Peanuts* cartoon. The last straw for his mother was when Danny dumped all of his dirty and very smelly gym stuff in the living room just as the members of the local flower club were arriving for the monthly meeting. After yelling and pleading to no avail, she decided she had to do something different. She bought a book by Gerald Patterson, called *Families*, and she read about positive reinforcement. She then used the following procedures to change the way Danny took care of his stuff.

First, she needed a positive reinforcer. Because Dan loved desserts, she decided not to fix any desserts until he took care of some of his junk in the hall. After 3 days, Danny finally hung up his coat when he came home. His mother immediately said, "How nice you hung up your coat. I think I will fix a cake for dinner tonight. Maybe you could pick up a few of your things from around the house." Dan did without being nagged. For the next few days, Dan was his normal self, and there were no desserts. Finally, he hung up his coat and took some books and clothes up to his room, and that night his mom served his favorite dessert (German chocolate cake and French vanilla ice cream). Over the ensuing weeks, Danny began to keep his stuff picked up and each night he did, there was dessert. At the end of about a month, his mother posted a list of things that should not be left lying around, on his door. Each day before dinner, she would check the house. If it was picked up, there was dessert; if not, no dessert. Occasionally, things were dropped or forgotten, but a brief reminder was sufficient to get them taken care of. Because his mother didn't have to yell at Dan any more (at least not about his junk), they got along much better.[3]

3. Some students have objected to this example because they felt that Danny was being manipulated by his mother; a person should have the right to be messy if they want and how come the teenager is always wrong? Was Danny manipulated? Manipulation usually implies deception and coercion. Neither of those occurred in this example, but the ethical issues involved in changing your own behavior and that of others are complex. These issues are discussed in detail in Unit 19, "Applying Behavior Analysis Skills with Others." Concerning the second point, in principle I agree that if a person wants to be a slob, he/she should be free to be one. However, it is seldom that a person has total freedom of action. We live in cooperative situations in which each of us places voluntary constraints on our actions for the good of the whole. Danny's messy behavior was very upsetting to his mother. As a consequence, she was often negative toward him in other situations. By changing these behaviors, a point of friction was removed, leading to their getting along better. This idea of reciprocity is also discussed in Unit 19. Finally, the teenager is not always wrong, but neither is the adult. It would be impossible to discuss solving everyday problems without considering the possibility that you or I are making mistakes that contribute to the problem. An important step in problem solving is recognizing our own errors so they can be corrected.

This story illustrates two major aspects of positive reinforcement.

1. You need a positive reinforcer that the person is relatively deprived of; that is, the stimulus (positive reinforcer) is not freely available to the person anytime he/she wants it.

2. The reinforcer needs to be delivered immediately after the response occurs. Here, it was sufficient to tell him immediately that there would be dessert tonight. Thus, his mother was able to select a *positive reinforcer* (dessert) that was not freely available and deliver it *immediately* (the same day), when the response occurred.

Positive reinforcement is a very important process that influences our daily lives in many ways. The people that we like are typically persons who give us lots of positive reinforcers. Similarly, we probably positively reinforce our friends' responses more than other people. The positive reinforcement can be as simple as smiling and saying how nice a friend looks when that person says hello to us. For most people, a smile and praise are positive reinforcers that will increase the frequency of that person saying hello to you in the future. On the other hand, positive reinforcement can involve more complex social or physical interactions such as helping someone with that night's homework or fixing dinner for mother. It is likely that you can think of many such instances of positive reinforcement in your interactions with family and friends.

Remember, positive reinforcement is a process that has been experimentally proven to be effective in increasing the frequency of responses in both the basic research laboratory with animals and in real-life situations with humans. As Danny's mother discovered, positive reinforcement can be more effective than nagging or yelling. And it is a whole lot nicer. We will talk more about positive reinforcement and how it can be used to change behavior in later sections.

Negative reinforcement is a very difficult idea to understand because the name just doesn't sound right. The word *negative* is often understood as meaning bad, while *reinforcement* is usually thought of as good. How can something be both bad and good at the same time? The confusion can be eliminated if it is remembered that negative reinforcement is a scientific term that has a very precise definition. Here, *negative* means to subtract and *reinforcement* means to increase. So when a stimulus is *removed* (subtracted) contingent on the occurrence of a response, and the frequency of that response *increases* in the future, the process is called *negative reinforcement*. Perhaps some examples will make the process of negative reinforcement clearer. Suppose our rat is now placed in an experimental chamber that has steel rods running across the floor and mild electric current is run through the rods and subsequently into the rat. It is likely that the rat would try to get away from the shock. If pressing a bar turned off the shock, it is likely that the rat would quickly learn to press the bar. This is an example of negative reinforcement. The response of pressing the bar subtracts or removes the stimulus of electric shock (a negative reinforcer) from the rat's feet, and this in turn increases the frequency of bar pressing.

Negative reinforcement results in the organism escaping the negative reinforcer. That is, by pressing the bar, the rat was able to escape (get away from) the shock. We often engage in behaviors that can be labeled "escape responses." Usually we go to the dentist to escape the present or potential future pain of a toothache, not because the dentist is a fun person to visit. Going to the dentist when we have a toothache is negatively reinforced by the elimination (subtraction) of the pain. Escaping negative reinforcers can occur in social situations as well. For example, I may be talking to a friend in the hall when another person comes up. This person is a real bore. He constantly monopolizes the conversation and talks only about himself. In short, he is not quite as bad as a toothache, but talking to him runs a close second. Under those circumstances the response of saying I have to do something else (e.g., go to the bathroom, library, meet someone else), will be negatively reinforced because it allows me to escape that situation.

Although negative reinforcement is important in teaching us how to terminate or escape painful physical or social stimuli, it can lead to difficulties, especially in social situations. For example, Sara is studying in her room and her younger sister comes in and wants to borrow Sara's favorite record. Because she usually brings them back with big scratches on them, Sara says no. But instead of leaving, she hangs around and pesters Sara about the record. (How come she can't borrow the record? She will be very careful with it, honest; she just has to listen to it and if you don't let her, she'll never speak to you again, etc.) She goes on and on until finally just to get rid of her, Sara says, OK. This is an example of negative reinforcement also. Sara's response of saying yes was negatively reinforced because it removed the stimulus of her sister's pestering. But if you remember the examples of positive reinforcement, you should have noticed something else about this example. The younger sister's pestering behavior was positively reinforced. That is, it was finally followed by the delivery of the record. This means that while giving her the record may have stopped the pestering now, in the future when she wants something from Sara, she is likely to try pestering again.

Sometimes we all negatively reinforce other people by our behavior. Say, for example, you want your parents to drive you and a friend to a football game and pick you up afterward. When you ask, they say no and you become upset and run to your room crying, "They are mean, don't really love you, and never want to help you." You continue crying in your room, and finally your dad says, OK, he'll take you. Then everything is fine, but is it? Your dad has been negatively reinforced because you stopped crying or yelling, but you have been positively reinforced for behaving in this way. The positive reinforcement of this behavior means that it is more likely to occur again in the future. Unfortunately, in the long run, this is probably not a good way to interact with your parents.

The accompanying Ziggy cartoon provides a possible example of negative reinforcement. Explain what the negative reinforcer is in this situation.

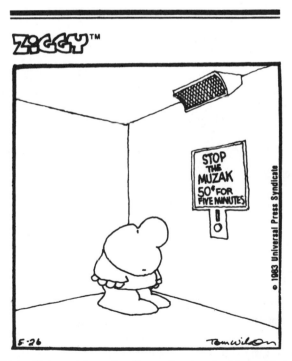

Study Guide

1. Reinforcement always _____ the
   probability of the response that produces it.

2. Positive reinforcement involves the

   _____ of a stimulus contingent
   on the occurrence of a response.

3. What stimulus did Skinner use as a positive reinforcer for the rat?

   _____

4. In general, for a stimulus to be an effective positive reinforcer, the

   organism must be _____ of it
   at other times.

5. For maximum effectiveness, the positive reinforcer should be de-

   livered _____ after the response
   occurs.

6. What behavior did Danny's mother change by using positive rein-

   forcement? _____

7. What method had Danny's mother used before trying positive rein-

   forcement? _____

8. Negative reinforcement involves

   _____ a stimulus contingent on
   the occurrence of a response.

9. Negative reinforcement results in a(n)

   _____ in the future probability
   of occurrence of the response that produced it.

10. A response that allows an organism to

    _____ a negative reinforcer will
    be more likely to occur in the future.

11. Situations involving negative reinforcement frequently also involve

    _____

    _____.

12. In escaping her little sister's nagging, Sara accidentally

    _____ reinforced the nagging be-
    havior.

UNIT 8

Punishment and Response Cost

The preceding unit discussed how consequences can be used to increase the frequency of a response. Sometimes, however, we wish to decrease the frequency of a particular response. You can also decrease a response's frequency by manipulating the consequences of the response in question. The major change from reinforcement procedures to punishment procedures is which stimuli are added or subtracted. Just as there are two types of reinforcement (positive and negative), there are two forms of punishment. But rather than calling them positive punishment and negative punishment (such labels become very confusing), we call the two forms *punishment* and *response cost*.

Procedurally, punishment is similar to positive reinforcement, with the obvious difference that it produces the opposite effect, a decrease in the frequency of the response. *Punishment* is the *delivery* of a stimulus contingent on the occurrence of a response that *decreases* the future probability of occurrence of that response. In other words, punishment adds a stimulus that results in a decrease in the strength of the response.

Response cost, on the other hand, involves taking a stimulus away. Procedurally, it is the same as negative reinforcement. *Response cost* is the *subtraction* of a stimulus contingent on the occurrence of a response that *decreases* the future probability of occurrence of that response. In short, whenever a response occurs, a stimulus that is already present in the environment is taken away, and the response then decreases in frequency.

Before discussing punishment and response cost any further, it must be noted that these are not pleasant procedures, and there may be general negative effects associated with their use. There are three possible negative side effects associated with these procedures. First, we tend to develop a dislike for people who use aversive procedures with us. For example, teachers who mainly use punishment in their classrooms are usually disliked by their students. Second, we try to escape or avoid negative reinforcers or aversive situations (remember the analysis of negative reinforcement). It follows that we would learn to escape or avoid people who use punishment or response cost a lot in their interactions with us. The converse is also true: If we use these techniques a lot, people will try to avoid us—even our friends. Finally, a person may react to punishment by trying to hurt the other person either physically or emotionally. For example, someone may try to change my behavior by making a nasty remark whenever I emit a particular response. But instead of changing, I may hit that person or say something even worse to him/her. Clearly, the result of trying to change behavior by punishment can be quite negative. Persons who are punished tend to dislike the punisher, try to avoid the punisher, and/or become more aggressive. As a consequence, even though we are presenting the scientific evidence concerning punishment and response cost, we certainly recommend that you *do not* use such techniques in your interactions with other people. These procedures should only be used by experts in situations that demand such drastic actions.

In punishment, the stimulus added is a negative reinforcer. Remember that negative reinforcers are stimuli that an animal or person will work to escape or terminate. Negative reinforcers strengthen behaviors that subtract the negative reinforcers from the person's environment. If a response produces or is followed by a negative reinforcer, it is logical that the animal or person will stop making that particular response. Recall, for example, the rat pressing the bar when it terminates an ongoing shock. Now, if pressing the bar produces a shock instead of subtracting the shock, it would take a pretty stupid rat to keep pressing the bar. In fact, under these conditions, the rat will quickly stop pressing the bar. The bar press then would be an example of a response suppressed by punishment.

Because of the negative side effects (dislike, avoidance, aggression), punishment isn't used as often as positive reinforcement in most therapy situations. But punishment can be a very important procedure when there are responses that must be eliminated for the health or well-being of the person making those responses. A case in point is self-destructive behavior. For some reason, some children occasionally develop behavior patterns in which they beat *themselves* until they do actual physical harm (black eyes, bloody noses, broken noses, and much worse). It's a terrible sight to observe a child doing this. As a consequence, most self-destructive children are physically restrained or given powerful drugs that tranquilize them. It is obvious that such children can't live normal lives under these conditions.

Dr. Ivar Lovaas, working with some self-destructive children, developed a punishment procedure to eliminate these responses. Lovaas used a painful but not physically damaging electric shock as the punishing stimulus. When a boy would start to hurt himself, Lovaas would say "no" and deliver the shock. After only three or four shocks, the boy stopped hitting himself. This procedure has proven to be a very effective treatment for self-destructive behavior and now makes it possible to work with these children without their being restrained or drugged. Punishment has been used in other therapeutic situations with good success in treating gravely serious problems. Thus, there is good evidence to support the use of punishment as a clinical tool, but again, we do not suggest you try it.

Response cost is another procedure that may be used to reduce the frequency of a particular response. Here, a positive reinforcer is taken away contingent on the occurrence of a response. Say, for example, that George's father pays him for doing certain jobs around the house each week. Money is a positive reinforcer for most people, and because George always seems to need money (in other words he is deprived of money), it is clearly a positive reinforcer for him. George and his father get along very well except for George's swearing. His father decides he will take away $.50 of George's allowance each time he hears George swear. Procedurally, this is an example of response cost; when George swears, he loses $.50 of his allowance. If George's father is consistent and George cannot earn money anywhere else, George will probably stop swearing in his father's presence. There could be difficulties though. For example, George might start fighting with his father about whether the fines were fair; if he is fined too much, George may just stop working, thus causing another fight with his father. In short, unless great care is taken, the response cost procedure might cause more problems than it solves. Just like punishment, response cost is best left to the professionals to use.

Response cost procedures can be very effective in institutional or group settings where they don't interfere with important interpersonal relationships. For instance, a community center was trying to run a recreation room where adolescents could come and play pool, ping pong, pinball, and other games. Unfortunately, the youths were very sloppy, and by the end of the day the room looked like it had been trashed. The adolescents were asked to keep the room clean, then threatened, and so on, but nothing seemed to help. Finally, it was decided that the director would check the room randomly on the average of every 30 minutes. If there was any trash anywhere in the room, the youths would have to leave and the room was locked for the rest of the day. The next day, the youths continued to trash the place, so the director made them leave and locked the room. The kids were very angry, but the director simply repeated the rule and left. The next couple of days were very hard on the director, but he continued to enforce the rule. Finally, by the end of the week, the youths started making sure that everyone took care of his or her own garbage. As a consequence, the recreation room stayed clean and open. From this example, you should be able to see how response cost should work. When you discuss this procedure with your teacher, be prepared to explain the following:

1. Why it was important that the director did not argue with the youths and consistently enforced the rule.
2. How the rule was an example of a response cost procedure.
3. How punishment and response cost are different.
4. Why it is probably a good idea not to try punishment or response cost procedures yourself.

Study Guide

1. Punishment and response cost are procedures used to

_____ frequency of a response.

2. In punishment, a negative reinforcer is

_____ contingent on the occurrence of a response.

3. In response cost, a positive reinforcer is

_____ contingent on the occurrence of a response.

4. List the three possible negative side effects of using punishment or response cost.

a. _____

b. _____

c. _____

5. Lovaas used electric shock to punish the

   _____ behavior of self-destructive
   children.

6. Taking money away contingent on the occurrence of a response is an
   example of what procedure?

   _____

7. What did the director of the community center do to reduce the
   amount of trash and litter in the recreation room?

   _____

UNIT 9

Extinction and Time-Out from Positive Reinforcement

In the preceding unit, punishment and response cost were shown to be effective ways of reducing the frequency of a response, but it was also argued that these procedures should only be used by professionals. What should a person do if a friend constantly emits a particular annoying response? Attempts at punishment would likely only produce negative reactions on the part of the friend. Fortunately, there is a less dramatic method of reducing the frequency of a response called extinction. In describing the Skinner and Greenspoon experiments, we have already covered extinction, but we did not call it that. *Extinction* is simply discontinuing or stopping the contingent reinforcement. When you conducted the Greenspoon experiment and the experimenter stopped following plural nouns with "mmhum" or "uhuh," that was an extinction procedure. Verbal approval is usually a positive reinforcer that strengthens the response it follows. When that approval is no longer given, the response that used to produce it gets weaker. Similarly, in the Skinner experiment, when pressing the bar was no longer followed by the delivery of food, the rat stopped pressing the bar.

Surprisingly, sometimes even negative attention such as criticism can function as a positive reinforcer. For example, the psychologist Wesley Becker worked with a group of teachers who were having discipline problems in their classroom. He found that the teachers' efforts at punishment (yelling at the class or individuals, criticizing, or ridiculing) actually seemed to increase the frequency of disruptions in the classroom. Becker then reasoned that the teachers' negative attention might actually be a positive reinforcer for the students (i.e., getting the teachers' goats). If that were the case, then having the teachers ignore the disruptive behavior might actually weaken it by extinction. In addition, Becker had noticed that these teachers did not praise their students' good behavior very often. So he told them to not only ignore the bad behavior, but to also frequently praise good behavior. Much to the teachers amazement the procedure worked; appropriate classwork increased in frequency and disruptive behaviors decreased. Interestingly enough, both the teachers and students seemed to be a whole lot happier. The procedure just described is called *extinction* and the *reinforcement of incompatible behavior*. *Incompatible* simply means that it is physically impossible to do both responses at the same time. For example, a person cannot smile and frown at the same time. In the Becker experiment it was assumed that a student could not work math problems and throw paper airplanes at the same time. If the amount of time the student spent doing math problems increases, there is less time to make and throw airplanes. So, by reinforcing the students' working on math problems and ignoring their throwing paper planes, it was possible to accomplish the goal of improved classroom behavior.

Extinction and reinforcement of incompatible responses are a very effective way of reducing the frequency of undesirable responses; unfortunately, people seldom use them. These procedures require thought, but when something another person does bothers us we often react immediately. That is, we try to use punishment or response cost because we can't think of anything else to do. In the accompanying example, Michael's dad did just that. Although Michael went to bed, how do you think he felt later?

Again, a better approach for dealing with a child who refuses to go to bed is extinction. Children frequently cry, argue, and throw temper tantrums at bed time, and parents similarly argue, threaten, and spank, usually without much effect. As a consequence, bedtime becomes a battleground for the family. Rather than arguing with the child, the parents should establish a bedtime rule. The child is then sent to bed or put in bed if necessary and those other behaviors of crying, arguing, screaming, and so on are ignored. If the child leaves the bed, he/she is simply put back in bed with a minimum of fuss. Several experimental studies of this procedure have been conducted. Each study has produced similar results. At first, the children are very resistant and cry for long periods of time, up to an hour, then gradually crying reduces to where they are simply going to bed. When the children were going to bed appropriately, the parents reinforced that behavior, and soon bedtime was a positive rather than a negative period. Extinction usually follows that course. First, the behavior increases in frequency and intensity and then it declines to zero or near zero.

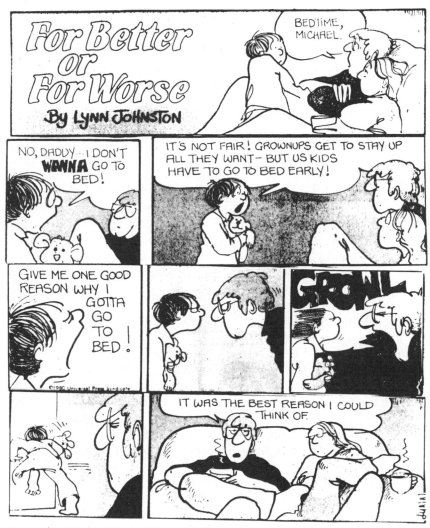

In summary, if reasonable care is taken, extinction is a procedure that anyone can use. It is simply a matter of not reacting to responses that bother you. Remember that the Becker study and many others have shown negative attention, criticism, arguing, and so on, often function as positive reinforcers that actually strengthen the undesirable response. But with a little thought, you can tell when something like that is going on. Then, instead of continuing to reinforce these behaviors with your attention, you can use the procedures of extinction and reinforcement of incompatible behaviors. In this manner, you can positively change the way your friends interact with you and vice versa without getting into "dumb" arguments.

The following example illustrates such a use of an extinction procedure in everyday life.[4] Mary was new to the school this year, but she seemed to be making many friends. She often met with one group of students during the lunch period. She had a nice time with them, and they liked her except for one habit: She consistently interrupted the conversation, particularly when Sally was talking. Mary always had something interesting to say, however, so they would pay attention to her interruptions. Sally finally became very angry with Mary for interrupting her all the time. She asked Mary to stop doing it, and Mary apologized and said she would stop. But, not surprisingly, she didn't. So Sally told her feelings to the others. They all agreed to ignore Mary whenever she interrupted Sally. Sally was to continue to talk and the others would simply pay attention to her and ignore Mary. However, when Mary contributed to the conversation at the right time, they did listen. Reinforcing the appropriate behavior is important. Otherwise, Mary might have simply stopped joining their group all together. After several lunch periods, Mary completely stopped interrupting Sally and everybody else as well. Also, the other members of the group seemed to like her even better now. The next unit describes an experiment designed to give you some experience using extinction and reinforcement of incompatible behavior to change another person's responses.

A procedure that is often used instead of extinction is *time-out from positive reinforcement*. A time-out procedure was used in the case of Ruby described in the first chapter. Remember when Ruby hit her little brother, she had to sit by herself in the dining room and do nothing for 5 minutes. This procedure had the effect of eliminating Ruby's hitting behavior. Time-out has elements of both *extinction* and *response cost* in it, but it is clearly different from both of them. In time-out, the behavior is not ignored as in extinction—something is done to the person. Unlike response cost, however, it is not a positive reinforcer that is taken away; it is the *opportunity* to earn more positive reinforcers that is taken away for a *specific time period*. There have been many experiments with pigeons on the effects of time-out, but a very clear example is found in a study of college students doing math problems. The math problems were fairly simple—two digit addition and subtraction operations. The students

4. Adapted from L. K. Miller (1980). *Principles of everyday behavior analysis.* Monterey, CA: Brooks/Cole. p. 89.

worked at a small computer and received a point for each correct answer and nothing for errors. The points could be exchanged for money after the experimental session. Under those conditions, the students worked very fast, but they made lots of errors. Next, a time-out procedure was instituted where the computer simply shut off for 1 minute after each error. This meant that the students were unable to work problems and earn points. After only half a session the error rate dropped to zero or near zero for all students. Notice that this is not a response-cost procedure because the points the student had already earned were not taken away.

Similarly, time-out differs from extinction in that something is actually done contingent on the occurrence of the response. In extinction, *nothing* happens following the response. For example, both time-out and extinction have been used to control the disruptive behaviors of retarded individuals during language training. Some developmentally delayed children do not learn to speak, so they must be given special language instruction. Usually, this consists of the individual and the speech therapist working intensively daily for about an hour at a time. The child can earn positive reinforcers (points, prizes, praise, food, etc.) for making correct responses, Unfortunately, the children often exhibit behaviors (e.g., playing with their hands, babbling) that interfere with the language instruction. Extinction has been used such that the therapist simply sits and waits until the child stops these responses before going on with the lesson. This procedure works, but it is very slow. The alternative time-out procedure works much faster, but it is somewhat harder to do. Just as the computer shut off for a minute when the students made errors, the therapist functionally shuts off by turning his/her back on the child when inappropriate responses occur. That is, when the child misbehaves, the therapist turns away, and the child can not earn any positive reinforcers for 1 minute. If the child is still misbehaving when the minute is up, the therapist simply turns away for another minute. This procedure is very effective in reducing the frequency of inappropriate responses. Time-out from positive reinforcement has proven to be a very useful procedure because it is faster than extinction but not as aversive as punishment or response cost.

Study Guide

1. Extinction simply involves no longer delivering

_____ reinforcers contingent on
the occurrence of a particular response.

2. Attention often functions as a

   _____ reinforcer.

3. One way of extinguishing a response (extinction) is to

   _____ it.

4. Many studies have shown that even

   _____ attention can serve as a

   positive reinforcer.

5. The teachers in the Becker study used

   _____ and the reinforcement of

   _____ behaviors to reduce the

   frequency of disruptive classroom behavior.

6. Give an example of a pair of incompatible responses.

   _____ and

   _____

7. How did the group reduce the frequency of Mary interrupting Sally?

   _____

8. The technical name for time-out is time-out

   _____

   _____

   _____ .

9. In time-out, the person loses the

   _____ to earn positive rein-

   forcers.

10. What happened when the students made math errors during the

    time-out condition? _____

11. In time-out, instead of ignoring the child's disruptive behaviors, the

    speech therapist _____

    _____ for 1 minute.

UNIT **10**

A Demonstration Experiment Using Extinction and the Reinforcement of Incompatible Responses

The present study is an extension of the Greenspoon experiment you conducted earlier in the course. This time, you will be looking at two classes of verbal responses—positive and negative about a second person. Basically, what you will be doing is reinforcing positive statements and putting negative statements on extinction. In order to conduct the experiment, you will have to learn the following definitions and procedures. The section of a paper that describes the experimental procedures is called the "Method."

Method

Subject

Another student in the school will serve as the subject. This should be a person you like and spend quite a bit of time with. The person should not, however, be a member of your class.

Informed Consent

Before you can conduct an experiment with anyone, you need that individual's permission. For the person to be able to make a reasonable decision about whether to participate or not, you need to give him/her some information about what will happen in the experiment. In this case, it will be sufficient to tell the individual that you are going to be studying the way he/she talks. Reassure the person that you will not be doing anything negative and nothing will happen to embarrass him/her or make him/her feel bad in any way. Finally, tell the person that nothing special will happen to indicate when the experiment is going on so he/she shouldn't worry about it. If the person says yes under those conditions, then you are set to start the experiment. If he/she says no, do not try to talk him/her into it; simply ask another person.

Experimenters

The demonstration works best with two experimenters. One person will have primary responsibility for carrying out the reinforcement and extinction procedures. The second experimenter has the major responsibility of recording the occurrence of positive and negative comments as well as reinforcing and extinguishing those behaviors.

Dependent Measures

Positive statements about others consist of verbal comments about a person not present at the conversation that point out some good feature or action. For example, "George really looks nice in his new sweater"; "Sally sure is smart, she got a 100 on the math test"; "Jeremy played well in yesterday's soccer game"; and "I like the way Julie is wearing her hair" would all be scored as positive statements.

    Negative statements about others consist of comments pointing out bad features or actions of a person not present at the conversation. For example, "Did you see George's new sweater? His taste in clothes is the worst"; "Sally certainly is dumb, she flunked her math test again"; "Jeremy really is a rotten soccer player, did you see him fall over the ball yesterday"; and "Boy, Julie sure got one of the ugliest haircuts I've ever seen" would all be negative statements.

    Remember that not all comments about another person have to be scored as positive or negative; they could be neutral. Statements such as "Mary went to the movie last night" or "Sara has to work after school" are simply observations that are neither positive nor negative. **If you have doubt about whether a statement is positive or negative, don't count it.**

Procedure

Extinction has been described in detail in the previous unit. For this experiment, the extinction procedure will consist of ignoring (doing nothing) in response to the negative statement and breaking eye contact for a brief period of time. When we speak to another person, we usually look at the person. This attention often functions as a form of positive reinforcer. During the extinction procedure, when the subject begins to make a negative statement, simply look away, look at the desk, the wall, over the subjects shoulder, and so on, until the statement is over and the subject is talking about something else. Then you can again look at the subject and make eye contact. Do not make any comment or argue in any way with the subject about the negative statement; simply ignore it. You should continue the conversation as if nothing had happened.

You will *reinforce* positive statements about another person by attending to the subject when they make such comments. Suppose the subject says, "Mary certainly looks nice today." The experimenter should follow that response with a positive comment about the subject, such as "Yes, she does, and I like the way you have your hair today," or "That's really nice of you to say so," or a simple expression of interest such as "mmhm," or even a smile and good eye contact. All of these consequences can function as positive reinforcers. If you use a mix of them, it is likely that some of them will serve as positive reinforcers for your subject.

You should begin the experiment by collecting a *baseline record* of how often the subject makes positive and negative statements about other people before you do anything. The baseline will consist of two 10-minute sessions held on consecutive days. The two experimenters should meet with the subject in casual settings, such as the lunch room, outside—someplace you might ordinarily meet and talk. You can talk for longer than 10 minutes, but the experimenter in charge of collecting the data should only record positive and negative statements for 10 minutes.

After collecting the baseline data, the *experimental condition* will be instituted the next day. Again, get together in a comfortable location and talk. But now the experimenter(s) will attend to and show interest when the subject makes a positive comment about another person and break eye contact and generally ignore the subject when he/she makes negative comments about another person. The conversation can continue for more than 10 minutes, but the second experimenter will only record data for 10 minutes. Implement the experimental condition for two sessions.

Data Analysis

To analyze the results of your experiment, make two graphs—one for positive statements and one for negative statements. Compare baseline levels of each response to the levels found in the experimental condition. Theoretically, if everything worked properly, the frequency of positive statements should have increased during the experimental condition and the frequency of negative statements should have decreased in comparison to the baseline. Remember, when analyzing your data, you are comparing the frequencies of responses found in the *experimental condition* to those observed during the *baseline* and not to each other.

Once you have made your graphs and discussed the results with your instructor, write a brief report describing what you did and why the procedures did or didn't work. Remember that it's just as important to notice why something didn't work as to know why it worked.

Behavioral Effects of the Basic Contingency Operations

The following definitions and table are presented as a review of the major conditioning procedures discussed in this book. By using this information, you can determine how a procedure should work and what effect it should have on behavior.

1. *Positive Reinforcement*: A *positive reinforcer* is *added* contingent on the occurrence of a response, and the future probability of that response is *increased*.

2. *Punishment*: A *negative reinforcer* is *added* contingent on the occurrence of a response, and the future probability of that response is *decreased*.

3. *Response Cost*: A *positive reinforcer* is *subtracted* contingent on the occurrence of a response, and the future probability of that response is *decreased*.

4. *Negative Reinforcement*: A *negative reinforcer* is *subtracted* contingent on the occurrence of a response, and the future probability of that response is *increased*.

5. *Extinction*: A response no longer produces a positive reinforcer, and that response *decreases* in future probability of occurrence.

6. *Time-Out from Positive Reinforcement*: A response is followed by the loss of the opportunity to earn positive reinforcers for a specific time period, and that response *decreases* in strength.

The following table summarizes the preceding definitions. The combinations of stimulus, operation, and effect are presented in this way to help you remember the major contingency operations.

Stimulus	Operation	
	Add	Subtract
Positive reinforcer	1. ↑	3. ↓
Negative reinforcer	2. ↓	4. ↑

↑ = increase in the frequency of the response.
↓ = decrease in the frequency of the response.

UNIT 11

Shaping

Psychologists have long been interested in how people acquire the responses they exhibit. Have you ever wondered how people learned some unusual behavior or skill? How does a person learn to juggle, ride a unicycle, or for that matter learn how to do long division, or how to drive a car? It should be fairly evident by now that the principles of reinforcement, extinction, and punishment are important in learning behaviors. However, in all of the previous discussions of these principles, the responses in question were already occurring. That is, before the reinforcement, punishment, or extinction procedure was applied, the behavior had already occurred. Remember what you did in the two experiments conducted so far. In the first, plural nouns were reinforced, but you waited until the subject actually said a plural noun. In the experiment, you did not teach the person to say plural nouns; the frequency of saying plural nouns was increased by reinforcement. Similarly, in the second experiment the frequency of positive and negative comments were changed, not by teaching new responses, but by changing the consequences of the existing behaviors. In many situations, behavioral procedures are used to modify the frequencies of behaviors that are already occurring. There are, however, times when it is necessary to actually teach new behaviors. This unit concerns one way to teach new behaviors, called "shaping."

Shaping is a process that produces new responses. Shaping is difficult to describe or define in the abstract, so we begin with a couple of examples. Jackson and Wallace[5] devised the following shaping program to teach a 15-year-old mildly retarded girl to speak loudly enough to be heard. Alice was diagnosed as extremely shy and withdrawn at age 7; she had no social skills, no friends, and learned little in school. A striking

5. See D. A. Jackson & R. F. Wallace (1974). The modification and generalization of voice loudness in a fifteen-year-old retarded girl. *Journal of Applied Behavior Analysis, 7,* 461–471.

feature of her behavior was that she spoke in a soft whisper that usually could not be heard. Jackson and Wallace, using very sensitive electronic equipment, differentially reinforced Alice for whispering one-syllable words appearing on a card in front of her. They continued to slowly increase the loudness requirement as she mastered each stage, until she was reading the words in a normal tone of voice. The investigators then went through a series of additional steps, including having her say things to other people, and so on. Jackson and Wallace also undertook a series of steps to help Alice transfer her newfound voice loudness to the classroom situation. After this training, Alice changed quite dramatically. She talked with other kids, she did quite well in a normal classroom, and she obtained a job as a waitress.

You can see the basic ideas involved in shaping from this example. A goal is set regarding a person's *target behavior*. In this case, the goal of Alice's target behavior consisted of getting Alice to speak in a normal voice with everyone she met. Next, the individual is observed to determine which responses currently occur. Before shaping, Alice always whispered. If you had tried to reinforce Alice's loud talking it probably wouldn't work because she would never have made a response you could reinforce. But she did whisper, and she occasionally whispered a little louder than usual. When she did, the louder whispering was reinforced. The louder whisper was called an *approximation* of the *target behavior* of normal talking. Once the loud whisper had been established, you could wait for an even louder whisper (a second approximation). This process involves the *extinction* (ignoring) of soft whispers and only reinforcing the louder ones. This combination of extinction and reinforcement is called *differential* reinforcement. Each new requirement is a *successive approximation*.

Shaping can occur accidentally. A person doesn't have to sit down and plan on shaping someone else's behavior; it may just happen. In addition to occurring accidentally, shaping can also produce undesirable responses as well as good ones. For instance, you could *accidentally* teach (shape) your parents to yell at you a lot. Say you are involved in some activity (reading, watching TV, or playing a game) and your mother calls. Usually you answer the first time, but this time she has to call again and louder before you answer. Because your answer is probably a reinforcer for your mother, you have just reinforced her for loud calling. The next time she calls, it is likely to be a loud call, and if you don't answer, she will call even louder. If the process continues, soon the call will become a yell. You have gradually taught (shaped) your mother to yell at you by only answering when she called louder and louder. Similarly, parents sometimes shape bad or inappropriate behaviors by ignoring

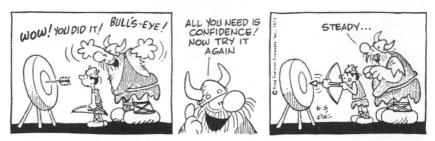

When using *shaping* to teach someone a new skill, you should start by differentially reinforcing behavior that the person can do successfully. Reprinted with special permission of King Features Syndicate.

their child's good behaviors (appropriate responses) and attending to them when they are behaving badly. It is quite possible if you think about your own experiences you can remember something like this happening to you.

Shaping, however, can be a very useful procedure. Perhaps there is someone with whom you would like to become friends. You could shape his/her friendly behavior. Does that sound odd? It shouldn't. Many psychological theories of friendship are based on mutual reinforcement. Just as shaping often occurs by accident, most of our friendships develop to a certain degree by accident, but that does not mean they always have to happen in that manner.

For the sake of example, let us say there is a girl named Joy you would like to get to know better. You know she occasionally smiles and says hello, but she never really stops to talk. Your first approximation to frequent long talks and other activities would be a short conversation. Shaping, of course, requires a reinforcer so the first step consists of finding a positive reinforcer or set of positive reinforcers for Joy's behavior. It so happens that most people enjoy being smiled at, asked questions about themselves, and complimented. You could try one or all of these. Now Joy smiles and says hello; you should smile in return and perhaps ask her a question about her classes. After she answers, smile again and say, "Have a nice day." Do not try to accomplish too much on the first interaction; remember you are just trying to get her to stop and talk to you.

After you are regularly having brief talks with Joy, add another question or compliment to the conversation (interaction). Gradually increase the length of conversation, using your smiles, compliments, and personal questions to reinforce her responses to you. Remember, if she fails to respond in turn you have to ignore her and only reinforce the behavior you want. Next, suggest doing something more extensive together (e.g., having a coke, attending some activity, visiting after school). Use your imagination to think of other possible activities. You should now have the basic idea of how you can use shaping to get a friendship started. Friendship, obviously, is much more complex than the example we have described. Whether you become good friends will depend on many factors such as the discovery of shared interests. On the other hand, the steps described could easily lead to the establishment of a long friendship.

In order to better understand the basic ideas of shaping, you should carefully read the following story. When you finish, some questions may help you analyze the example.

Mary was a very shy girl who hardly ever talked to anyone. Several people, including her teachers, noticed her problem. They all decided to help her. The decision was made to be nice to her every time they saw her talking to another person. Unfortunately, Mary's talking behavior did not change at all. The teachers decided that they needed some advice about how to help Mary with her problem. So they consulted a psychologist who suggested a different method for getting Mary to talk.

The psychologist told the teachers that for Mary, talking to other people would be a new response (one that she currently cannot do). The psychologist decided that first of all, the teachers should begin by asking Mary very simple questions that required only a "yes" or "no" answer, such as "How are you?" "Did you enjoy class today?" "Are you going home now?" If Mary answered the teachers, they were to reinforce her by smiling and saying it was good to talk to her. If you did not answer, the teachers were to just walk away.

When Mary was answering the teachers' simple questions more often, the psychologist had the teachers ask questions that required more than a "yes" or "no" answer. For example, they were to ask Mary, "What did you learn in class today?" "What did you do last night?" "What are your plans for the weekend?" Again, if Mary answered, the teachers would smile and thank her for talking to them. If she did not answer, they were to walk away and say nothing. In addition, if Mary answered "yes" or "no," the teachers were to ignore that answer and ask the question again.

Once Mary began giving longer answers to questions more of the time, another step was introduced. The teachers were now instructed to have Mary ask them questions. The teachers asked Mary to ask them something. One teacher asked Mary to ask about what the teacher was going to do the next day in class. Or to ask what the teacher was going to do after school. Again, Mary was reinforced for asking the questions and ignored when she did not.

Soon, the teachers began noticing that Mary was talking and asking them questions. At first, talking and questioning did not occur at a high frequency, but with frequent praise, talking and questioning increased over time. The teachers also noticed that the behaviors had *generalized*, and Mary was talking more to the other students as well as with them.

1. In the story about Mary, what procedure was used?

   _____

   a. What was the target response?

      _____

   b. What successive approximations were used?

      1) _____

      2) _____

      3) _____

      4) _____
   c. How was differential reinforcement used?

      _____

2. Why do you think that in the beginning the teachers could not get Mary to talk by being nice?

   _____

3. Were the reinforcers used by the teachers effective? _____
   What is the evidence for your answer?

   _____

4. Why do you think Mary found it easier to talk to the other students after the teachers helped her?

   _____

In order to really understand an idea or set of ideas, you must be able to use it in a new situation. Instead of giving you another example of shaping for you to analyze, choose a response that you would like to teach to another person or an animal. Specify the target response. Next, suggest several approximations of the target response.

1. The target response is _____.

2. The approximations are

   a. _____

   b. _____

   c. _____

   d. _____

   e. _____

3. Describe how you will use differential reinforcement to shape the new response.

   _____

Study Guide

1. Reinforcement, punishment, and extinction are all important to _____ behavior. However, these procedures only increase or decrease the frequency of a response. They cannot produce a _____ response.

2. Shaping is a procedure used to produce a

   _____

   _____.

3. The specific behavior that is to be produced is called the

   _____.

4. The small steps that are involved in shaping procedures are called

   _____

   _____.

5. Differential reinforcement involves the use of

   _____ and

   _____.

UNIT 12

Stimulus Control: Discrimination

Up to this point, the analysis of behavior has focused on the effects of consequences on responses. Consequences are, of course, stimuli that follow responses, but other stimuli influence how a person responds in a particular situation. If these stimuli precede the response, they are called "discriminative." A *discriminative stimulus* (S^D) is a stimulus that *precedes* a response and *indicates* that reinforcement is very *likely to follow* that specific response. This sounds like a very complex definition, but it is really quite simple. If you make a particular response in the presence of a discriminative stimulus for that response, reinforcement will usually follow. For example, Tommy has learned that if his mom is smiling when he goes into the kitchen, the response of asking for a cookie frequently will result in his mother giving him a cookie. (We know, in fact, that other variables such as how close it is to dinner will influence whether Tommy gets the cookie, but for the sake of a simple example, we will ignore those factors right now.) In this case, his mother's smile is the discriminative stimulus for the response of asking for a cookie.

How did the smile become a discriminative stimulus? Stimuli become S^D's through a process called *discrimination training*. Discrimination training involves the reinforcement or extinction of a response depending on whether a specific stimulus is present. The example of Tom's mother's smile can be represented as follows:

Stimulus	Response	Consequence
Smiling mother	Asking for a cookie	Cookie
Frowning mother (not smiling)	Asking for a cookie	No cookie

Our behavior is influenced by antecedent (before the event) discriminative stimuli (S^D's) when different consequences for a particular response is possible. Sometimes, when Tommy asked his mother for a cookie he got one, and other times he did not. Over a number of tries at asking for cookies, he learned that the times he got a cookie were the times his mother was smiling when he asked. If she was frowning, no cookie. Very quickly Tommy learned to ask for cookies only when his mother was smiling. Mother's smile has now become a discriminative stimulus for Tommy's response of asking for a cookie because it indicates that Tommy probably will get a cookie if he asks now and not at some other time when she is not smiling.

Examples of discriminative behavior are an important part of our everyday lives and thus are present almost everywhere. For instance, consider a person wandering around a large building trying to get out. If she were to find a door marked "Exit" and go throught it, she would be reinforced by the consequences of getting out of the building. If, on the other hand, she were to go through doors marked "Men" or "Librarian," she would not be reinforced, because aside from anything else that might happen, she would not have gotten out of the building. Thus, as a function of the process of learning to recognize discriminative stimuli (S^D's), doors marked "Exit" will become discriminative for the response of leaving the building.

Basically, we learn to use words in this manner. A clear example that the use of words involves a discrimination process can be seen in the way a child learns to call only one particular person "mother." At first, the parents are excited about the child's efforts to say words they understand and reinforce all approximations of the word "mother," whenever the child makes one. As a consequence, the child learns to say "mother," but he/she may then use the name incorrectly when mother is not there or apply the name to some other woman who may be present. Because we usually do not want children calling all women "mother," the parents begin only to reinforce the response "mother" when the child calls one particular woman "mother" (i.e., his/her mother). When the child calls another person "mother," that response is extinguished or corrected. Quickly, the child learns to use the word "mother" only in reference to that one particular person; that specific person is now an S^D for the response, "mother."

Discrimination is a very important factor in determining our patterns of social interactions. Not surprisingly, people become discriminative stimuli for the responses that they reinforce. That is, if one person tends to reinforce "silly" responses, and another reinforces "serious" responses, we will act differently (silly or serious) when we are with one person and not the other. This process of discriminating how other people reinforce us was demonstrated in a study with preschool children. There were two experimenters who would alternate coming into the free-play period of the preschool day. One experimenter consistently reinforced the vigorous active play of the children (tag, wrestling, playing with large blocks, etc.) and ignored quiet playing, whereas the second experimenter reinforced quiet playing and ignored active play. Very quickly, the children learned to discriminate between the two experimenters. They then played actively in the presence of the first and quietly when the second experimenter was present. You and I make the same sort of discriminations. We talk very differently when we are with our parents than when we are alone with friends our own age.

Thus far, all of the examples we have discussed have involved positive reinforcement. However, a stimulus can also become discriminative for negative reinforcement. Remember, negative reinforcement involves emitting a response that removes or subtracts an unpleasant stimulus, and because the response removes that stimulus, its strength is increased. The basic experimental research on this process is called "discriminated avoidance." In an earlier unit, the example given to explain negative reinforcement involved research with a rat that pressed a bar to escape electric shock. When the shock came on, the rat had to press the bar to turn it off, and the rat quickly learned to do this. But the environment can be arranged so that the rat can avoid the shock altogether. To do this, a warning stimulus indicates that the shock is coming. In this way, instead of pressing the bar to escape the shock, the rat can now press the bar to prevent the shock from being turned on. Say for example, a tone is sounded 10 seconds before the shock is turned on; if the rat presses the bar, the tone goes off, and the shock is not presented at all. The rat becomes very good at pressing the bar as soon as the tone comes on because otherwise it will receive a shock. The tone has become a discriminative stimulus (S^D) for the negative reinforcement (removal or prevention of shock) of pressing the bar.

Does this sequence remind you of anything that happens in your everyday life? People frequently give warning signals. Sometimes the signals are subtle, such as a frown; at other times, the signals are loud and clear, such as yelling or slamming a door. These signals usually indicate that we had better make some response or a negative reinforcer will quickly be delivered (i.e., punishment). The response may be in the form of escape or avoidance (e.g., when mom or dad really slams the door coming in the house, a good response is going to our room and reading).

On the other hand, some particular response may be required, and the warning signal indicates that it is time to emit the response, or a

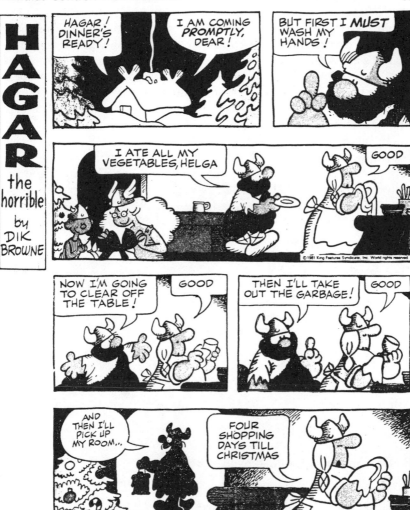

Responses that have been reinforced during particular periods or in specific situations in the past become very frequent when those conditions reoccur. Reprinted with special permission of King Features Syndicate.

negative reinforcer will be delivered. For example, it may be your responsibility to set the table for dinner. The announcement that it's time to set the table would then be a discriminative stimulus for the response of setting the table. The response of setting the table is negatively reinforced because it prevents the presentation of such stimuli as a yelling father or mother, the loss of allowance or privileges, and so on.

Just as people can become discriminative stimuli for positive reinforcement, they can become discriminative stimuli for negative reinforcement as well. We tend to avoid people who are obnoxious or boring. If I find George to be that type of person, and I find out that he will be here in a little bit, I will probably try to leave the setting. We are making those sorts of discriminations when we are invited to a party and we ask, before accepting, "who is coming?"

In summary, discriminative stimuli precede responses and indicate that reinforcement is likely to occur if a particular response is made then. Our ability to learn the relations between discriminative stimuli and the reinforcement of particular responses is crucial for our everyday social interactions. If we are sensitive to those cues, we are better able to get along with the people around us.

Study Guide

1. Antecedent stimuli that affect the frequency of a response are called

   _____

   _____.

2. Discriminative stimuli come to influence responses through the process of _____

   _____.

3. Discrimination training involves both

   _____ and extinction of the same response in the presence of different stimuli.

4. When Tommy's mother was smiling, the response of asking for a cookie was _____.

5. For a child to learn to call only one person "mother," the response, "mother," to all other people must be

   _____.

6. A stimulus can become a discriminative stimulus for

   _____

_____ as well as positive reinforcement.

7. A discriminative stimulus for negative reinforcement can also be
   called a _____ stimulus.

8. A person can become a _____
   _____ for the response he or she
   reinforces.

9. Why did the preschool children engage in active play when one
   experimenter was there and not when the other experimenter was
   present? _____

   _____

10. Discriminative stimuli _____ re-
    sponses.

11. Analyze the accompanying Garfield cartoon in terms of the dis-
    criminative stimulus for negative reinforcement. In other words why
    did Jim act the way he did when Garfield got on his chest?

    _____

Reprinted by permission of United Feature Syndicate, Inc.

UNIT 13

Stimulus Control: Generalization

Generalization refers to a person making an *old response* in the presence of a *new (novel) stimulus*. For example, when we meet new people, they sometimes resemble (look like) people we already know. If a person reminds us of a very good friend, we are likely to behave nicely and positively toward the new person. If, on the other hand, the person reminds us of someone we dislike, then we may act unfriendly or coldly toward this individual. The responses to the new person are an example of generalization. They occur, not because of anything the new person has done, but because as a stimulus, the person is similar to someone else we know.

The process of generalization is based on past discriminations. Responses to new situations or novel stimuli occur because of the past consequences for responding in the presence of similar stimuli or situations. For example, the child's verbal response, "dog," is based on a generalization of responses to similar animals in the past. It also involves a discrimination between the stimulus set of dogs and that of all other animals. The discrimination training will involve having the child apply the name "dog" to one particular animal, such as the family dog, and not to another animal, such as the family cat. The family dog is then an *example* of the group, set, or class of stimuli, dogs.

As the child is reinforced for calling this animal a dog, generalization of the naming response to other similar animals will occur. The first generalization will be related to the most obvious features of the family dog, such as size, color, hair length, and so on. So if the family dog is small with long grey hair, the child may call Aunt Martha's large grey long-haired cat a dog. The negative feedback for this response ("No, that is a cat") will teach the child that other features are important in determining whether an animal should be called "dog." Similarly, upon seeing a Saint Bernard or Great Dane for the first time, the child may not know what to call it. After a few more experiences such as these, the child will learn that dogs come in all sizes and shapes and are distinguished (different) from cats and other similar animals by some common physical features and general behavior (e.g., dogs bark; cats meow). As a consequence, the child will be able to identify correctly new animals as dogs or cats. From this examination of how a person learns to tell dogs from cats, it should be clear that generalization and discrimination are closely related.

Although we have focused the discussion on the generalization that occurs when we meet new individuals or animals, generalization is an extremely important part of our responses to new situations as well. For instance, you are invited by a friend to stay over Saturday night and spend Sunday with her. You find Sunday's activities include attending worship service with your friend. Because you and she have different religious affiliations, how do you know how to act at the new religious service? Because we assume here that going to a worship service is not a totally new situation, generalization could occur from your similar past experiences. Responses that have been reinforced at worship services in the past will probably be acceptable here. Also, you friend is available as a model of correct behavior. Finally, you would discriminate the differences between this worship service and other worship services and other settings where group activities occur, such as a basketball game. While there are similarities between the setting of many religious services and a basketball game (each involves groups of people; they both may be held in large buildings; and in each there may be major players or participants and others who observe or participate in a different way), these similarities are not important for determining what behavior is appropriate in that situation. You must discriminate both the similarities and the differences in order for correct generalization to occur.

Failure to discriminate differences as well as similarities can lead to generalization errors. A generalization error can be as simple as the child calling a cat "dog," but they can have far more serious implications. For example, when you say to a friend or to yourself "This guy looks like a wimp, loser, jerk," or other name, you are making a generalization. You are either consciously or unconsciously deciding that persons who look like this also behave in ways I don't like; therefore, I will not like this person.

But you could be making an unfortunate error that could cost you a potential new friend. Just as it is difficult, if not impossible, to tell whether an animal is a dog, based on the fact that it has four legs, it is equally difficult to tell if someone would be a good friend based on one or two features, such as the person's size or the way they dress. After making derogatory remarks, you may later discover that the guy you called a "wimp" is actually the most popular boy in the school because he is kind, generous, and goes out of his way to help people. You may have messed up the chance to be his friend by automatically generalizing the response wimp, because he resembled someone you didn't like in the past.

The admonition, "Don't judge a book by its cover," refers to the fact that appearances do not always predict worth. Or to phrase it in the terms of this unit, don't generalize on the basis of too little information. When people act in haste or on impulse, they are usually making a generalization error. Such behavior can lead to serious consequences, such as losing a friend or getting into a fight with parents. A good rule of thumb is to consider all aspects of a situation before acting. In this manner, you are more likely to correctly discriminate and generalize so that you can then engage in the appropriate behavior.

Study Guide

1. Generalization involves making an

   _____ response in the presence

   of a _____ stimulus.

2. Generalization appears to be based on the

   _____ between old stimuli or

   situations and the new stimulus.

3. Generalization also involves

   _____ training.

4. In teaching a child to identify dogs, the family dog is an

   _____ of the group of stimuli

   called dogs.

5. In order to correctly generalize, you must discriminate both the

   _____ and the

   _____ between the old stimulus

   situation and the novel stimulus situation.

6. Failure to discriminate _____ in
   stimuli can result in generalization errors.

7. Do not _____ on the basis of too

   _____ information.

UNIT 14

An Experiment in Discrimination Training

The preceding units described discrimination and generalization training and how they affect behavior. In this study, the experimenter attempts to establish a discrimination based on the idea (concept) of *male*. The experiment is adapted from a procedure developed by Professor Israel Goldiamond of the University of Chicago. The study shows how discrimination and generalization are involved in the way we learn the meaning of words.

Method

Subjects

One or more other students will serve as subjects for the study. They should be people you know and whom you are fairly sure will cooperate. One fun way of increasing the participation of the subjects is to offer a reward at the end of the experiment if they get the last three questions right. The reward could be a soda, candy bar, small prize, or just a favor. The reward needn't be very large; it is just used as a way of increasing the subjects' incentive to learn the discrimination.

Experimenter and Observer

One experimenter and one observer are needed to conduct this experiment. The experimenter will have the responsibility for presenting the stimulus materials and telling the subjects which response is correct. The observer will record which response is made by which subject before the experimenter announces the correct response.

Materials

The following list of stimulus pairs will be used to teach the discrimination. The positive member of each pair is called the discriminative stimulus for the concept. The discriminative stimulus is *followed* by an ×. The subject should select this stimulus.

	Left	*Right*
1.	A	B (×)
2.	B (×)	D
3.	O	B (×)
4.	JB (×)	AQ
5.	URB (×)	VOX
6.	BULL (×)	COW
7.	SOW	BOAR (×)
8.	BUSTER (×)	NANCY
9.	DAISY MAE	LI'L ABNER (×)
10.	ROBERT (×)	MAY
11.	BOY (×)	GIRL
12.	ROY (×)	GAYLE
13.	ANNETTE	RODNEY (×)
14.	HEN	ROOSTER (×)
15.	SONNY BOY (×)	LISA
16.	RITA	ROB (×)
17.	ALBERT (×)	BETSY
18.	EDNA	WILLIAM (×)
19.	LOUISE	GEORGE (×)
20.	EDWARD (×)	RACHEL
21.	JOHN (×)	ROBERTA

The subject will need an answer sheet. This will consist of the numbers 1 through 21, followed by the choices left and right. Plain notebook paper can be used to make the answer sheets, but they should look something like this:

1. Left _____ Right _____
2. Left _____ Right _____
3. Left _____ Right _____
4. Left _____ Right _____

    .
    .
    .

21. Left _____ Right _____

Procedure

The observer should first pass out the response sheets to the subjects. Then the experimenter should explain to the subjects that stimulus pairs will be presented and they are to choose one of them as correct. The subject will then write the stimulus selected next to the left or right alternative on the response sheet. The experimenter should also explain that there will be a pattern in the stimuli that the subjects should be able to identify at the end of the experiment.

   The experimenter will then present the first set of stimulus pairs. After all of the subjects have *written* down their answer, the experimenter will announce which response is correct. If a subject selects the wrong stimulus, have them cross off the wrong response and then write in the correct one before continuing.

   After the subjects have responded, but before the experimenter has announced the correct response, the observer will make a tally mark on his/her record sheet to indicate how each subject responded. For example, if there are four subjects and three chose the left stimulus and one the right, the observer's record should look like this:

1. Left ——————— III ——————— Right ——————— I ———————

   At the end of the experiment, the observer should have a complete record of all of the subjects' first choices for each of the stimulus pairs.

   After all of the stimulus pairs have been presented, the experimenter will ask the subjects to write what they think is the reason why one response is correct. The experimenter will then explain that the discriminative stimuli were all associated either with the concept of male or contained the letter *b*, with *male* being the primary discrimination stimulus. If the subjects meet the criterion for the reward, they should be given the reward at this time. Finally, the experimenter should thank everyone for their participation and ask if there are any questions.

Data Analysis

After the experimental procedure is completed, the observer should graph the results. The graph will consist of the percentage of correct responses for each stimulus pair. For example, if there were four subjects the graph should look similar to the graph at the bottom of this page. (That is, if only one subject of the four were correct, the graph would be marked at 25%.)

In analyzing the graph, the observer and experimenter should look for stimulus pairs where the percentage correct was 50% or less. If there are places where accuracy was that poor, then there is a problem with the training program.

In addition to the group responses, the individual responses should be examined. If a subject makes the wrong response to two or more stimulus pairs in a row, this also indicates a problem in the program.

Finally, the subjects' written ideas about why one response was correct and not the other should be analyzed to see whether they actually learned the concept of male.

After the analysis has been completed, discuss with the instructor both the results of the study and ways to improve the program.

Conducting this experiment should give you a better idea of how discrimination and generalization are important in every aspect of our lives. Also, you should have a better idea of how we learn concepts or ideas.

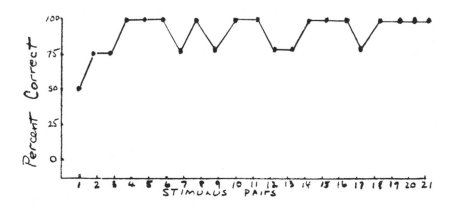

UNIT 15

Observational Learning: Modeling, Imitation, and Identification

Do you ever wonder why some styles of clothes or sayings are very popular for a while and then disappear, only to be replaced by the latest rage? This process of changing styles or fashions is not new. A look at a well-illustrated history book or a series of photo magazines covering 5 or 10 years will show a steady change in what persons wore during that time. Even a cursory review is enough to prove that these changes did not always make the clothes more comfortable or functional. For example, during the Elizabethan period in England, men of prominence or importance wore a strange arrangement of ruffles that stuck out from their waists. These ruffles were very clumsy, collected dirt, and had no function other than high fashion. Women in the "Gay Nineties" (i.e., 1890s) went to another extreme to produce stylish waists. They wore corsets that constricted their waists to such abnormally small sizes that it was dangerous to their health (fainting was very common and frequent). Again, there was no reason for our female ancestors to endanger their lives except for style, high fashion, and the like.

Similar changes can be seen in the way we talk, especially in that area of language called slang. When I was in high school, you did not simply say "no" in answer to a question. Our response was the rhetorical, "Do elephants pole-vault?" Presumably, this was meant to convey the meaning, "no." To me, there is still something pleasing about that phrase. Perhaps it is the vivid image I have of the pole snapping as the poor old elephant is just getting off the ground. Nonetheless, our parents did not find this response to be a particularly appropriate (i.e., a wisecrack). So around them, we tried (not always with success) to remember to simply say, "no." More recently, a whole new language evolved and flowered in California called "Valley Girl Talk." Most of the country only adopted a few quaint phrases such as, "Gag me with a spoon," but for a time in Southern California, it was possible to find yourself in situations where you did not know the language even though it sounded like English. But this, too, is now considered passé or old.

What does all of this have to do with psychology or self-management? There are really two issues here. The first has to do with the psychological principles involved in the development of such odd behaviors by so many people while the second concerns how such trends affect our own behavior. In the first case, we are likely to explain these trends or changes in fashion as fads, but calling them fads does not explain why they occur. Why should a large number of people start wearing their hair shorter, longer, or purple; lengthen or shorten their skirts/pants or buy flowered skirts/blouses instead of checked ones? The term *fad* or *trend* is simply a name or label for these phenomena. The question of why people go along is not answered by saying it is a new fad. People simply do not catch a fad like they catch a cold or the flu. Instead, fads or trends are part of a much larger set of psychological phenomena that have been variously labeled "modeling," "imitation," and "identification." We review the basic ideas about these processes because they have subtle but important effects on all of us and our actions.

Although in theoretical psychology there are some major differences between modeling and imitation, they are not important for us now and are not discussed here. A great many experiments have been conducted on imitation, but the basic ideas are quite simple. One child observes a second engaged in some task. The second child (the model) completes the task in a particular way (e.g., placing a set of blocks in a required order) and is then given a reward such as a toy or a piece of candy. The observing child is next given a chance to play with the blocks, and she too places the blocks in that order and is given a reward. This is an example of learning by imitation.[6] The first child observed the model respond and be rewarded, then she imitated that response (did the same thing) to earn a reward for herself. The main components of imitative learning are a model, an observer (imitator), the demonstration of a novel behavior, and the apparent availability of reinforcers for making that response.

6. Note that the term *imitation* as used here is a scientific one and not derogatory. Frequently, when we say something is an imitation, we mean it is fake and not very valuable because it is not real. The behaviors involved in imitation are in fact valuable and real; the term *imitation* simply refers to the way in which they were learned.

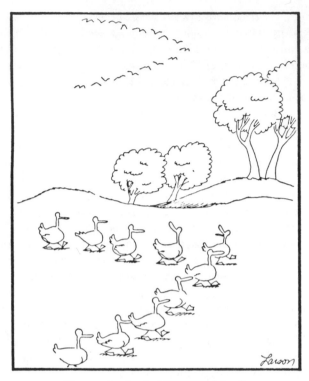

"Say . . . Look what THEY'RE doing."
Sometimes we learn valuable new skills by imitation. *The Far Side Cartoon* reprinted by permission of Chronicle Features, San Francisco

This simple set of psychological variables can become very complex and can have profound effects on our lives.

A good time to observe the development of behaviors by imitation is when young children (2 or 3 years old) are really learning to talk. As they are expanding their vocabularies, they mimic (imitate) the new words they hear other people say, television commercials, and phrases from the latest hit songs. These are examples of verbal imitation, and in this way, children can easily learn many new words. Because we all imitated verbal stimuli as children learning to speak, it is not surprising that later in our lives we find ourselves unconsciously imitating popular phrases or sayings. Thus, the fads we talked about earlier can be seen to be the result of our tendency to imitate new, different, or salient (catchy) responses. Interestingly enough, we are not alone among the animals in terms of imitation; other primates such as macaques, chimpanzees, and gorillas all imitate. To date, no one has observed any groups of these animals long enough to determine whether they also have fads, but it would not be very surprising if they did.

Some further examples of imitative fads are when you see a particular hairstyle modeled by a famous person become popular with all of the girls you know; or all of the boys start wearing jerseys that a famous football player or team wears. You should now recognize that many advertising campaigns are designed to work based on imitation. Cigarette and liquor advertisements in particular show people in exciting, glamorous, and/or romantic situations. The model smokes a specific brand of cigarette and is rewarded by having something happen to him/her that the rest of us would like to experience. Obviously, you are supposed to believe that if you use this particular brand of cigarette, these wonderful things will also happen to you. In scientific terms, the advertisers hope you will imitate the model's responses and buy their product. Of course, we know that just because we smoke one brand of cigarette, males will not become macho cowboys with beautiful women attracted to them and females will not magically become liberated or glamorous. But we may believe it a little bit—just enough to buy those cigarettes.

All of the commercials that appeal to you by showing someone using their product and then being rewarded by fame and fortune are hoping that you will unconsciously or unthinkingly imitate the model in the advertisement. If you sit down and analyze what is being shown in the commercial, it is clear that the product they are trying to sell has almost nothing to do with the actor, what he/she is doing, and what happens to the person. Of course, many good products may be advertised in this way, but the advertising has nothing to do with the relative value of the product. You should only buy a product after carefully evaluating in an unemotional manner whether or not it is what you need and not because the commercial promises you love and happiness.

We have discussed in detail how imitation works in advertising because the same processes occur in other situations. We are likely to become involved with the characters in films or television shows because of all the exciting and dramatic things that happen to the protagonist (hero/heroine of the show). We may then imitate some of that character's more interesting responses. Again, this is one of the ways that fads often begin. Imitating a TV character's behavior, however, is not always a good thing to do. Research has consistently demonstrated that school-aged children, adolescents, and adults will respond more aggressively after watching a violent television program than after watching a comedy.

Although we will not immediately go out and hit someone after watching *The A Team* or become devious and vicious from being a fan of J. R. in *Dallas*, the things we see (observe) can affect our behavior.

Sometimes, imitation of a particular person goes beyond wearing the same sort of clothes or hairstyle as a particular person to talking the same way, favoring the same foods, drinks, cars, and so on, and in general mimicking their mannerisms and lifestyle as much as possible. When imitation is so complete the process is called *identification*, and the person who does the imitating is said to have *identified* with the second person or model. In identification, it is psychologically important to become as much like the model as possible.

Many psychologists think that when we are young, we identify with our same-sex parent (i.e., girls with mother and boys with father) as a way of *vicariously* experiencing the power that our parents seem to have. *Vicarious* in this context means feeling rewarded or reinforced by someone else's accomplishments or behavior as though they were our own. So, even though we do not have the ability to make a particular response, by identifying with father or mother we can also feel rewarded when they are. For example, young children often play house and pretend to do the things they see father or mother doing. If you observe young children carefully, usually everyone wants to be an adult (father, mother, the police officer, etc.), while the youngest child gets stuck as the baby or the family dog. Obviously, babies or dogs, even when playing house, do not get to do the same sorts of exciting things as adults.

As we get older, other people frequently replace our parents as the primary models for how we behave and think about ourselves. On television, in magazines and newspapers, and through other sources, we are presented with the details of the lives of rock musicians, TV and film stars, athletes, fashion models, and prominent women and men in politics, science, and the arts. We are attracted to these people because of both their accomplishments and the rewards they are seen to be enjoying. We want to be like the star performer not only because of the skill the performer displays but also for the applause the person receives. We can also come to identify with a person through personal contact. We may admire an older brother or sister, the family doctor or lawyer, a favorite teacher, or a friend's parent for the person's accomplishments, lifestyle, or possessions. There are many possible reasons for identifying with and imitating the behavior of another person, but usually the people we choose seem to be happy, to enjoy what they're doing, and to feel satisfied with life.

In identification, our vicarious satisfaction of another person's success is increased when that person is like us in some way. The greater the similarity between myself and the person with whom I identify, the more I enjoy this person's success. It then follows that I can increase my vicarious satisfaction or pleasure in another person's success by changing myself to be more like the model. By identifying with another person in that way, we often make very important changes in our behavior without thinking about it or even recognizing why.

However, identifying with a person who has developed great skill and accomplished important goals can be a good way of setting goals for ourselves. We may wish to be like a particular actress, politician, writer, or scientist because we admire what that person has done. The person's actions, and lifestyle appeals to us because they are similar to what we would want to be and how we want to live. When we have such goals, it helps give direction to our lives. For instance, if you want to be a writer like a famous author you admire, there are a number of basic skills you must develop because without them you cannot write. Similarly, to be an actress, musician, or athlete, there are essential skills, techniques, and so forth, that you must acquire. To acquire those skills, you must learn more about acting, writing, or whatever; then you must put yourself into a position to learn those skills (apprenticeship program, college, various schools, etc.); then you must practice those skills until you finally may succeed. Thus, in deciding to become a doctor because you identify with a particular doctor, his/her skills, and role in society, you have determined many of the important things you must do in your effort to become a physician. In short, identification is an extremely powerful process that can have a profound effect on your life.

Study Guide

1. Odd trends of fashion in language are called

   _____.

2. Fads develop as a function of

   _____

   _____ and

   _____.

3. When one person learns a new response by watching another person,

   it is an example of _____.

4. Young children often _____
   things they hear in TV shows or movies.

5. Many advertisements are designed to get you to buy the product in
   order to _____ the models in the
   commercial.

6. Sometimes, imitation can have negative effects, such as when people
   imitate the _____ they observe in
   programs.

7. What is a more extensive form of imitation called?

   _____

8. What does vicarious mean?

   _____

9. How is identification important?

   _____

Starting a Fad—"Do Elephants Really Pole-Vault?": A Demonstration of the Power of Observational Learning

The objective of this exercise is to introduce a new slang term into your school—one that you invent so that you can be sure that it has never been used before. The procedures of modeling and reinforcement will then be used to introduce your slang into the school by starting an imitative fad. The exercise is not an experiment because there will be no control procedures or nontreatment control group. Nevertheless, because of the unique content and objectives of the project, it should be quite clear that the procedures are responsible for starting your fad.

Method

Subjects

The rest of the student body of your school will be observed for changes in their verbal behavior. Because it is not an experiment and the procedures will only directly involve your class, it is not necessary to formally ask the other students to participate. Your class will simply observe to see if the frequency of the slang saying you invent increases in use in the school.

Project Managers

Because the exercise will be going on outside of class for at least 2 weeks, it is necessary to select two students who will coordinate the procedures. Their responsibilities will be to make sure that the models and reinforcers are trained and then carry out the procedures in the appropriate manner. The managers will also assign observers to various parts of the school and collect and analyze the data.

Experimenters

There will be two groups of experimenters. The first will be the models. The students chosen to be the models should be very active in school affairs and very outgoing—that is, comfortable talking to other people. The second group of experimenters will be the reinforcers and secondary models. These students will at first be responsible for praising and showing interest when a model uses the slang term and then after about 3 days they will start modeling the phrase also. In order to get the fad going, you will need at least six primary models and six reinforcers. Both of these groups of experimenters should be made up of equal numbers of males and females and should reflect the ethnic balance of the school.

Observers

The rest of the class members will work on the important task of data collection. The task of the observers will be to listen and record whenever the slang phrase is used by someone in the school other than members of your class.

Stimulus Materials

The first thing that needs to be done for this project is to think up your own slang word, term, or phrase. This will be trickier than it sounds because for you to be able to analyze your results the word or phrase must be completely new to your school. One method of producing the slang for your project would be to look at old magazines in the library. Both the stories and the advertisements from 20 to 25 years ago should provide examples like "Do elephants pole-vault?" and "Dig you later alligator," a snappy phrase that meant "Good-bye." Alternatively, it might be more fun and challenging to create your own. Whichever method you use, the slang needs to be catchy and short so that your models can use it a lot in their conversations. The easiest forms of slang to use are substitutes for "yes" or "no" and adjective phrases such as bird-brained, lead-head, dog-breath, and so on.

Modeling Procedures

The models and reinforcers will work in two-person teams of one model and one reinforcer. The model and reinforcer will work themselves into conversation groups (bunches of kids talking together) at lunch time, between classes, and after school. So that the procedures seem natural, they should not always arrive together. Sometimes the model should be the first to go in the group, and other times the reinforcer should. When they are both in the same group, the model will try to use the slang in the conversation. The reinforcer will then immediately call attention to the slang by laughing and/or making some comment about the slang such as "very clever, what did you say?" and so on. Only use the new slang two or three times in each conversation, otherwise your fellow students may think the model is simply weird or strange rather than remembering the slang. At first, these procedures will seem unnatural, so they should be practiced in class before trying them with friends and acquaintances. After about 3 days, the reinforcers–secondary models should start using the slang in their conversations, and finally in the 2nd week everybody in the class should use it off and on when appropriate. After 2 weeks, everyone in the class should stop using the slang.

Recording and Data Analysis

The data for this study should be very simple to collect. It is not necessary to collect detailed information on who used the slang or when.[7] Because the project is concerned with the demonstration of how a fad can start and spread, the observers need only tally when they hear anyone other

7. For some experiments on social psychological factors in group imitation, it would be important to record such information. In fact, you might wish to record whether the person who uses slang is female or male to see if there are any sex differences in the spread of your fad. I am sure you can think of many other bits of information that could be collected or variations in the procedures that could be run to demonstrate other factors in the relations between imitation–modeling and the development of fads. If you come up with a really good one, please write and tell me about it.

than a member of the self-management class use the slang. Although there should not be any baseline frequency of use of your slang term by other students in the school before the modeling begins, to ensure that this assumption is correct, the observers should begin their task of recording the use of the slang 2 days before the modeling procedure is begun. Data will then be collected for a 3-week period: the 2 weeks the modeling procedure is in effect and 1 week after it has been terminated. Data will be graphed and analyzed in terms of the daily frequency of the slang response. If the demonstration works correctly, there should be an increasing frequency of slang use by other students over the 2-week period. It is impossible to predict what will happen after the 2-week period. The fad may fade quickly or you may discover that you have started a nationwide fad something like the human "wave" cheer that became so popular at sporting events. However, unlike those people now claiming to have started that fad, you will be able to write to *Time* magazine and prove how you started this one in your class.

UNIT 17

Classical Conditioning: Fear and Anxiety

To this point, our study of behavior has focused on operant behavior and the principles involved in analyzing operant responses (e.g., discrimination and schedules of reinforcement). However, an important set of human behaviors appear to be developed in a different way—*emotional responses*. Emotional responses such as fear, anger, and love involve actions of the autonomic nervous system. Without going into technical detail, the autonomic nervous system (ANS) is that part of the central nervous system that controls the body's relatively automatic (at least, generally not consciously determined) reactions to pain, threat, stress, and the like as well as general body functions. The ANS functions on the basis of a variety of physiological responses that are biologically built into our bodies.

Although it does not involve emotion, a good example of such an ANS built-in reaction is the pupillary reflex. If you go into a dark room, your pupils (the dark center of your eye) automatically dilate (enlarge) to let in more light. In contrast, when you go out into the bright sunlight, your pupils constrict (get smaller) to let in less light. These adjustments are made automatically without your having to think about them. In fact, you usually have very little voluntary control over these responses. For instance, if I threatened to hit you if your pupils constrict when I shine a bright light in your eyes, you might try to close your eyes but you would not be able to prevent your pupils from constricting. Similarly, I might offer you $5.00 if you could make your pupils constrict when asked. Unfortunately, you probably would not collect because you can not make your pupils constrict simply by saying to yourself, "Pupils constrict."

Emotional responses, while they far more complex than these reflexes, are based on the same sort of built-in ANS responses. Emotions are conditioned reactions related to those ANS responses. Because emotions are based on conditioned reactions, before we can understand them, the ideas of classical conditioning must be examined. This form of conditioning was discovered by the great Russian physiologist–psychologist Ivan Pavlov. Pavlov worked on the salivary reflex of dogs: When dogs eat, they secrete large amounts of saliva (we do also, but not with the same gusto). Pavlov found that dogs would automatically salivate if he blew a small amount of meat powder in their mouths. Pavlov then did something very clever; he paired giving the dogs the meat powder with sounding a tone. Tones do not ordinarily make dogs salivate, but it was found that after a few pairings of the tone with the meat powder, sounding the tone alone would cause the dogs to salivate. He called the dogs' learned reaction to the tone a *conditioned reflex*[8] and the tone a *conditioned stimulus*. The following table represents what Pavlov did, and it should make the experiment easier to understand.

	Stimulus		*Response*
1.	Meat powder placed in the dog's mouth	— Elicits ——→ (automatically produced)	Salivation by the dog.
2.	Meat powder paired with tone	— Elicits ——→	Salivation by the dog.
3.	Tone alone	— Elicits ——→	Salivation by the dog.

The idea for Pavlov's experiment probably came from the common observation about people's reaction to the sight, smell, or even thoughts of food. Stop for a minute and think of your favorite food. It may be a thick and juicy steak, apple pie and ice cream, or a particular candy bar. Whatever it is, try to imagine what it looks like, how it feels, and how it tastes. After a few moments, most people will find that their mouths start to water (no doubt the basis of the phrase, "mouth-watering good"). Salivating after thinking about food is an example of a conditioned reflex.

Our reactions to telling ghost stories is another everyday example of a conditioned reflex. Here, if the story-teller is very good, we start feeling some of the physiological reactions associated with fear. A really scary story may be said to make the hair on the back of your neck stand.

8. Actually, Pavlov labeled them "conditional reflexes," but the term was translated as conditioned and that has been used in the West ever since.

Sometimes such phrases may be used metaphorically but other times our hair may actually stand up. This reaction is caused by our skin tightening, which in turn is caused by the ANS shifting blood from the extremities to the muscles and other organs important for us to be able to run from harm or to fight if we can't escape. How do these aspects of the ANS responses to pain become associated with ghost stories?

One of the first psychologists to systematically study the conditioning of fear was J. B. Watson. Watson tested hundreds of young infants and discovered what he labeled three basic emotional responses: fear, rage, and love. Fear was produced by either an unexpected loud noise or the loss of support. The infant's fear response was characterized by first a sharp intake of breath and then uncontrolled crying. The rage response was reliably elicited by restricting the infant's ability to move—that is, holding its arms close to the body. The infant would first struggle then become red in the face and start yelling—distinct from the crying shown in fear. Finally, the responses of smiling and cooing—what Watson called love—were produced by gently stroking the child's body. Watson argued that all of the later emotional responses that adults display were developed from these three basic unconditioned responses displayed by infants.

Whether Watson was correct is still a matter of debate in psychology. Nonetheless, Watson was able to demonstrate how fears can be developed or conditioned. In this famous study, he and Rosalie Rayner worked with a toddler named Albert. Albert was a healthy, chubby, phlegmatic child who did not appear to have any unusual fears. This was tested by placing a tame white rat into his playpen to see how he would react. Albert immediately approached the rat and started playing with it. This was done for several days to show clearly that Albert was not afraid of the rat.

Then one day, while Albert was playing with the rat, an experimenter snuck up behind Albert and struck two pieces of metal together producing a sharp, loud, and unexpected noise. Albert was startled and immediately began crying. The rat was removed and Albert was comforted.[9] The next day, the rat was again placed in the playpen, and when

9. It is appropriate to ask whether this was an ethical thing to do to a young child. My answer is probably no, but the issues are complex. Was Albert permanently harmed by these experiences? Again, this answer is probably no. You will learn about the extinction of conditioned fears, and it is likely that this fear extinguished naturally. In designing experiments involving humans, scientists consider what is called the "risk/benefit ratio" plus such factors as deception, coercion, and consent in trying to determine if an experiment is ethical. In Unit 19, the issues will be discussed in the context of your use of psychological procedures to change behavior.

Albert approached the rat, the loud noise was produced again. Not unexpectedly, Albert started crying. The next day when the rat was placed in the playpen, instead of approaching it, Albert immediately started crying and tried to get away from it. Notice that the loud noise was not used that day. The rat had now become a conditioned stimulus that could elicit the fear response by itself.

But that was not all. When a furry white stuffed toy rabbit was given to Albert, instead of playing with it, he pushed it away and started crying. It was discovered that not only white rats but any white sort of furry thing (even a white bath towel) would produce crying and other fearful responses. The fear response had generalized from the white rat to all stimuli similar to it in terms of color and fluffiness. The idea of generalization was discussed earlier regarding stimulus control and operant behavior. The process is essentially the same in classical or Pavlovian conditioning. Generalization refers to the situation in which a novel stimulus now produces a behavior previously produced by the stimulus used in the conditioning. For generalization to occur, the new stimulus must be similar in some way to the original conditioning stimulus.

From our perspective, Albert's fear of the fluffy white bath towel was unreasonable or irrational. That is, objectively, there was no good reason to be afraid of the bath towel. It had never been paired or associated with the fear-producing stimulus (the sudden loud noise). Thus, the study with Albert demonstrates not only how the fear of a particular stimulus can be produced (conditioned) but also how it can spread to other stimuli, creating inappropriate fears. The accompanying cartoons provide some humorous examples of conditioned fears, but of course, ordinarily such fears are not a laughing matter.

Another psychologist, Mary Culver Jones, was the first to demonstrate how such fears could be eliminated. She worked with young school-aged children who were extremely afraid of all animals (dogs, cats, rabbits, etc.) that they might normally have as pets. The procedure she used can be called counterconditioning. The idea was to associate or pair animals with pleasurable activities or stimuli rather than fearful ones.

The actual procedure Jones developed for doing this was a very clever and creative extension from psychological theory to practice. First, she tested the children with real rabbits to measure their reactions. All of them became very tearful, resistant, and distressed when the rabbit (clearly in a cage) was brought into the room, and if it came within 5 feet, they cried and tried to run away. She then observed them in the lunchroom eating and talking with friends and an adult helper. As lunch started, she placed a rabbit in a cage at the far end of the table to see if it

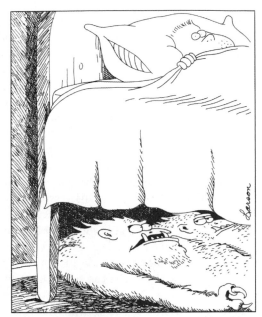

"I've got it again, Larry . . . an eerie feeling like
there's something on top of the bed."

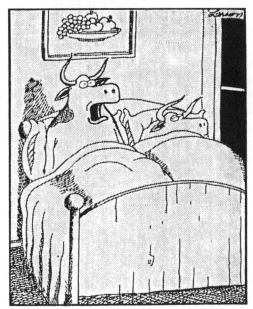

"The golden arches! The golden arches got me!"

The Far Side cartoons reprinted by permission of Chronicle Features, San Francisco.

upset the child (she only worked with one child at a time). The child barely noticed the rabbit and kept on eating and talking. Over the course of successive days, the rabbit was moved closer and closer to the child until it was sitting right next to her. The child was then asked to give it some food through the cage wall. Finally, the cage was left open, and the child asked to hold the rabbit. The procedure was successful with about 80% of the children, and their fear of other animals was reduced enough that they could be taught to play with them as well. So, although some fears are easily learned, they can also be unlearned.

Sometimes we may have a vague feeling of fear or unease that does not seem to be clearly caused by any particular stimulus, situation, or thing. This general feeling of unease and distress is one of the forms of anxiety. The second and most frequent form anxiety takes is that of a less intense or low-level fear related to a general class of events or situations. For example, I may say I have butterflies in my stomach or that I am nervous before giving a presentation at a conference of psychologists. I am not really afraid of giving my talk in the same way I would be afraid if I slipped while rock climbing. Nonetheless, I am uncomfortable and worried, and if asked would say I am anxious. Although anxiety is not as intense as fear, it can still disrupt our lives. When a person is anxious about a coming event, it becomes difficult to think about or to concentrate on other important activities. The person also will probably imagine and worry about everything that possibly could go wrong. The worry and concern then seem to make the situation even more aversive, causing even more concern, and so on. Finally, the focus on and worry about possible mistakes increases the probability that one of them will actually occur. This is because the person will think about these things in the actual situation and not about what the appropriate responses are.

Not surprisingly, for most of us, fear and anxiety are very aversive feelings or sensations.[10] Because they are aversive, we seek to terminate or avoid them and the situations that produce them. Recall that the termination or removal of aversive stimuli was described earlier as *negative reinforcement*. In negative reinforcement, a response that leads to the termination or removal of an aversive stimulus is strengthened or increases in frequency. Under most circumstances, learning responses that escape or avoid aversive or painful stimuli is a good thing. We

---

10. There appears to be a group of individuals for whom the intense body sensations associated with fear appear to be exciting and positive reinforcers rather than aversive. These individuals have been called "thrill seekers" by Garlington and actually seem to pursue danger. It is not that they do not feel fear but instead that they report enjoying it. These people sometimes have psychological problems because of their attraction to danger, but that is a topic for more specialized books.

probably would not survive very long if we did not! But sometimes, avoiding emotionally aversive stimuli or situations can lead to maladaptive and inappropriate behavior. Returning to the earlier example, if, instead of tolerating the mild anxiety associated with public speaking, I started avoiding such situations to escape the associated anxiety, that would be an undesirable result of negative reinforcement. If I never speak publicly about my research, others won't know about it, and my job wouldn't be done as well. Similarly, we often allow the mild anxiety about possible embarrassment associated with meeting new people, trying new dances, learning a new language, or trying out for the school play to keep us from doing those things even though we really want to do them.

What can a person do about these unwanted and undesirable effects of fear and anxiety? A few years back, Dr. Alan Gross and I helped some college students who were extremely afraid of white rats (I doubt that any of them had had steel bars banged while holding a white rat but they were afraid nonetheless). Although there are situations where it is appropriate to be frightened of rats, the white rat, for the most part, is a tame and harmless creature. These students, like the children in the Jones study, were unable to be in the same room with a rat without becoming very anxious and upset. Their problem was further complicated because many of them were psychology majors who would have to do experiments with white rats to finish their psychology training. They were helped to overcome their fears and anxiety through a self-management counterconditioning program.

Although each program was individualized for the particular student, the essential components of the program can be summarized as follows. First, the students were helped to analyze the problem as clearly as possible (i.e., what was it about white rats that made them anxious?). Second, they designed a series of steps or approximations to the target behavior, similar to the successive approximations used in shaping. Next, they selected a set of small rewards they would give themselves when they completed an approximation. This procedure ensured that the rat was being systematically paired with positive reinforcers or events. Finally, they were asked to actually carry out the approximations over the next 2 weeks at their own pace or schedule. The students were, however, cautioned that if they became upset during a step, they were to stop and go back to the preceding step and successfully complete it before continuing.[11] At the end of 2 weeks, the students were tested and all could now approach, pick up, and hold a rat for 30 seconds without becoming upset.

11. They were also told that if they had real trouble they should contact the experimenters; none did.

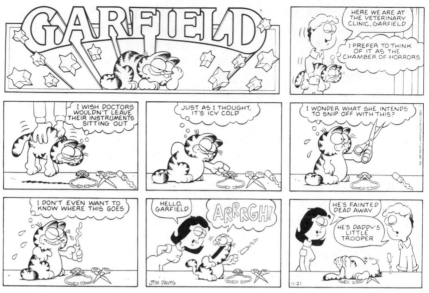

Reprinted by permission of United Feature Syndicate, Inc.

Variations on these procedures can be and have been used to deal with a wide range of difficulties related to fear and anxiety. The essential steps are analyzing the problem, deciding what you should do in the situation, figuring out some approximations to those behaviors, and carefully working through them while making sure that there are positive consequences associated with each. Certainly, it is often more difficult to deal with our fears than this summary makes it sound, but with some thought and effort, many of the fears that limit us can be eliminated.

Study Guide

1. Fear is an _____

_____ which is based on

_____

_____

_____ reactions.

2. In the pupillary reflex, the pupil automatically

_____ in response to bright light.

3. Pavlov paired a tone with

_____

_____ to make a dog salivate.

4. After the pairing, the _____
   alone could elicit the salivary response.

5. Hair standing up on the back of your neck during ghost stories

   is an example of a _____

   _____.

6. How did Watson elicit rage?

   _____

7. A white rat was paired with a

   _____

   _____ to produce a conditioned
   fear.

8. The fear then _____ to rabbits
   and white bath towels.

9. How was Jones able to eliminate the fear of animals? By

   _____.

10. What is a vague, general, low level fear called?

    _____.

11. Fear and anxiety can be very disruptive because we learn to

    _____ or

    _____ situations which produce
    them.

12. Summarize the Gross and Brigham procedures used to elimi-

    nate the fear of rats. _____

    _____

II

APPLYING BEHAVIOR ANALYSIS SKILLS

The first section of this book presented the basic principles and procedures of behavior analysis. Although those ideas were discussed in the context of everyday life situations and examples, it is now time to systematically examine how these procedures can be used to solve personal problems. The procedures and techniques presented in this section are drawn from the area of psychology called "applied behavior analysis," "behavior therapy," or "behavioral engineering." Scientists working in the area of applied psychology–behavioral technology publish their research in journals (science magazines) such as the *Journal of Applied Behavior Analysis, Behavior Therapy, Behavioral Engineering*, and the *Journal of Consulting and Clinical Psychology*, to name just a few.

The research reported in those articles is designed and directed by professional scientists, but a lot of evidence suggests that you and I can use many of those procedures to solve many simple problems of everyday living. So I took the main ideas from several of those articles and present them in a how-to-do-it fashion that should make them relate directly to common daily problems. This section also includes reports by students such as yourselves who have taken a course in self-management. These reports indicate how the student applied some self-management procedures to solve a personal problem. Finally, while we hope you will do a personal self-management project as a part of your course, you don't have to do a full study or project each time you have a problem in order for the procedures to be useful. Every day, we have opportunities to improve our lives by regularly using positive reinforcement, extinction, problem-analysis techniques, and so on, to solve or even prevent minor problems.

A Laboratory Case History

Sarah was a very pretty 10th-grade student—auburn hair, an attractive face and figure—and to most people the picture of an extremely attractive, vivacious, and intelligent young woman. Yet she had extreme behavioral problems at school, both with peers and with teachers. While a gifted student, Sarah had never received a report card with even average grades. She was in a high school class of approximately 120 students, and all the teachers knew her because of her disruptive behavior. As a result, Sarah made frequent visits to the administrative office and was, therefore, equally and similarly known by the secretaries, the principal, and her fellow students. Sarah also appeared to be a very unhappy person, perhaps partly because she had tried very hard to be friends with some of the students in her class and had not succeeded.

After exposure to the program described here, however, Sarah changed within 6 months to a student with a B average, who had not been referred to the administrative staff in the past 3 months, and who had a wide group of friends. (She had received 3 invitations to parties, 2 invitations to go to the movies, 14 invitations to go to football or basketball games, 2 invitations to slumber parties, and 65 invitations to visit a friend's home after school.)

Teachers made such comments about Sarah (after her participation in this project) as: "I can't imagine what's happened to her, but whatever it is, it's wonderful"; "She used to be constantly fighting with me, the other teachers, and the students, but now she's charming and delightful; she's now one of the most popular students in her class."

When Sarah was asked about what the project had meant to her, including the details of gathering the data and handing it in and learning specific interventions with peers, she gave the following interview:

I didn't get along with most of the other students very well back then, so he [Mr. Farrin] asked me if I would like to be in the program with him. At first I didn't know, but then I thought I might as well try it; at least I would get out of the classroom for part of the time.

One of the first things that I did was try to change a person's attitude against me. Mr. Farrin asked me to name three people with whom I wanted to make friends. They were Raphael, Jim, and Amy. Then he asked me how many times any of them say nice things about me. He also wanted me to carry a little card around with me and mark it down on the card. So I carried the cards around with me in my purse and marked down on a card every time the guys said anything nice to me. Then I'd sit down with Mr. Farrin and we'd talk about it. After 2 weeks we talked about how many ways we could increase the nice things they said to me.

We used a theory that every time Amy said something nice, I'd offer to help her with her work, or something similar to that. Or, if Amy complimented me on something, I'd compliment her back. Then for the first two weeks I ignored her if she said anything bad to me. But then, when she said anything nice to me, I'd help her with her work, or I sat down and asked her to do something with me, or something like that. That's the way it went pretty much.

Jim was the one that was always saying bad things about me. And for the first 3 weeks when he said something bad, I would just ignore him; I'd turn my back on him, like he hadn't said anything, or something like that. Then when I met with Mr. Farrin again, he asked me if I could think of anything to improve the situation with Jim so that he would quit saying bad things about me. I said "Well, I think if I keep ignoring him, it's going to be okay, because he doesn't say as many bad things about me anymore."

The first time that Jim ever said anything to me that was even nice, like even hello, or the first time he even walked by me without saying something bad to me, I gave him a great big smile and I said, "Hi, Jim, how are you today?" When I first did that, Jim looked like he was going to die. I guess I had never said anything nice to him before and you could see that Jim didn't know what to do with it when I said that. He was so surprised his mouth just opened and he looked at me and he couldn't think of anything to say. It took him so much by surprise that he didn't say anything bad to me for about 4 days. The first time I had a chance, I said to him, "Hi, Jim, what are you doing?" He was by himself then, and I was with a group of other kids, and I asked him if he would like to come over and talk with us for awhile. Again, Jim was so surprised he didn't know what to do, and he came over and talked with us and I smiled at him as nice as I could. Boy, I'll tell you the count on him really went down. He wasn't calling me any names at all. That's all it took with Jim. I just ignored him for awhile and then I was really friendly to him when he was nice to me and he's always nice to me now.

With Raphael, it was the same thing. It was how many times he would call me names. Raphael was always calling me names; in fact, Raphael calls everybody names. I don't think anybody likes Raphael. I'd write down every time Raphael called me a name and I'd take the cards into Mrs. Christenson, the school secretary, every day after school.

Then when I'd sat down with Mr. Farrin and talked to him again, we'd talk about all of the stuff we'd written down on the cards and how that was helping me and how everything was going. But Raphael was really a tough one. He'd always call me names when all of his friends were around and they would all laugh at me and so would he and he would just keep on doing it. They all thought it was really funny. So what I did, every time he called me a name, I just ignored him. But sometimes with Raphael, ignoring him didn't work because the other kids laughed and made Raphael want to do it more. The next thing I did was I would turn away and I wouldn't even look at him. I did with Raphael just like I did with Jim, but with Raphael I saw that if he was standing around with his friends I tried to stay away from him, because if he had some kids around that would laugh, he would always like to call you names so he could get the attention of the kids. So I knew with Raphael, if he had a bunch of other kids standing around, you had to stay away from him because he was going to call you names. But I waited until he was by himself and I walked up to him and I'd say, "Hi, Raphael, how are you today?" and I'd smile at him. He was just like Jim, he just didn't know what to do.

The first time, when I said, "Hi," he still called me a name, because he thought I was being mean to him. I guess that was because I'd never said anything nice to Raphael, although hardly anybody ever does. I guess the only way Raphael ever gets anybody's attention is by calling people names and being mean and fighting. But after six or seven times, when Raphael was by himself, I'd say "Hi," he'd kind of smile a little bit and I smiled right back at him. Then one time I was standing with a bunch of my friends again and Raphael came by all by himself. It used to be that anytime I was with any of my friends and Raphael came by—by himself—I'd call him names and poke fun at him and say, "Look at him with his curly head, look at that weird-looking guy." He isn't really very tall for a tenth grader; he's shorter than the rest of the guys, and he's very self-conscious about this. So when Raphael came by and saw me with my friends, I think he thought I was going to tease him, but I said "Hi, Raphael, how are you?" and one of the other girls said it too, and then we started talking to him and he came over and talked to us for awhile. At that time, we were going to go play some cards and we asked him to come along and play with us.

I think next year when I'm in eleventh grade, if I don't get along with the students very well, I'll need this and it's going to help me and I know how to use it and I know I'll need this theory like Mr. Farrin taught me to do. I don't think I'd use the card to mark things down anymore. I don't think I need it anymore, I can handle it on my own by just ignoring people, saying nice things to them, or asking them to do nice things with me that are fun, or helping them with their homework. I really liked knowing how I can make the students like me, or make them leave me alone. I never knew how to make friends.[12]

Study Guide

1. In this case study, Sarah, an attractive intelligent student, was having

   trouble at school because of _____

   _____ problems.

2. She also appeared to be a very

   _____ person.

3. The school counselor helped Sarah change her

   _____ and also how other people

   _____ toward her.

4. The first step was to pick out three students that Sarah would like to

   become _____ with.

5. She then recorded their _____ to
   her.

6. Next, she _____ bad comments

   to _____ .

12. This study was modified from P. Graubard & H. Rosenberg (1974). *Classrooms that work*. New York: E. P. Dutton. pp. 35–40.

7. Finally, Sarah used her positive social comments and help with homework to _____ their positive behaviors.

8. Raphael was especially difficult for Sarah to make friends with because of his continued name calling. What consequences were maintaining Raphael's negative responses?

   _____

9. How did Sarah deal with this problem?

   _____

   _____

UNIT 19

Applying Behavior Analysis Skills with Others

The use of reinforcement, punishment, extinction, and shaping have been emphasized in different situations in previous units. By this time, you should be able to define these procedures and know when and how to use them appropriately in dealing with brothers, sisters, parents, and especially your friends. The advantages of using these techniques to interact with others can be summed up in two ways. First, you will become more aware of your own behavior and the effect it has on others. Consider the effects your behavior has when you pay attention (a powerful reinforcer) to friends when they demonstrate inappropriate behaviors. Second, you should be able to use the procedures you have learned both to your advantage and to the advantage of others. Can you think of some occasions when you may have reinforced, punished, extinguished, or shaped the behavior of a friend without knowing it?

Graubard and his associates[13] did a study that helped some students who were having problems. Specifically these youths were having problems in school and had reputations as trouble makers. Much like Sarah, their behavior had resulted in their being unpopular and frequently ignored or reprimanded by the teachers and other students in the school. So the students were taught how to reinforce the teachers. They were instructed to smile at the teachers whenever a teacher talked to them or saw them around the school. Of course, the students now understood the reinforcement procedures, so they did not smile when the teachers were

13. See P. Graubard, H. Rosenberg, & M. Miller (1974). Ecological approaches to social deviancy. In R. Ulrich, T. Stachnick, & J. Mabry (Eds.), *Control of human behavior* (Vol. 3). Glenview, IL: Scott Foresman. pp. 421–431.

angry at them. The results of this procedure were very interesting. The teachers began paying more attention to the problem students and also looked at them more often during class periods. Also, while they reinforced the teachers, they also became more friendly with the other students who had the same classes. Do you think they could have been reinforcing the other students also?

The study demonstrated to the problem students the effects that their behavior could have on others. It also taught them how to use reinforcement to their advantage and probably to the advantage of the teachers and other students. Why these youths had problems in the first place in school is hard to say. It may have been that they were shy or that in the past their efforts at making friends were not successful, so the only way they could get attention was by being a trouble maker. A more likely reason why adolescents have problems dealing with teachers and other people their own age is that they do not realize how their behavior affects other people.

In psychology, the term *reciprocity* is used to label or name an interaction between two people in which each benefits. For example, you may help a friend with some math problems, and he/she in turn may help you repair your bicycle. You may not do both things right in a row or even on the same day, but over a period of time things will probably be pretty even. One way of identifying friends is whether they mutually reinforce each other. This common sense notion has been formalized in the theory of psychological equity sometimes known as "exchange theory." Basically, the theory suggests that in any exchange between two people or groups of people, the psychological gains or benefits and losses can be calculated (added up) for each party. For the exchange to be *equitable* or fair, the sum for one party must be approximately equal to the sum for the other party. If the exchange is unfair, the person or group that gained the least from the exchange will attempt to change the relationship. One way of changing a relationship is to end (terminate) it. Frequently, when people terminate an unfair relationship, bitterness and hard feelings are involved. That is, the ex-friends can end up fighting or yelling whenever they meet in the future. As the concept of reciprocity suggests, for a relationship between two people to be maintained, it must be fair, and they both must gain from the exchanges.

The idea of equity can be applied to any type of relationship between individuals and groups. For instance, when you buy something from a person or store, you are exchanging money for goods or services. If you like the product, you are likely to engage in future exchanges (buy something else) with that party. On the other hand, if there is something the matter with the product, you are less likely to buy there in the future.

It may seem odd to talk about interactions among friends, between parents and children, and among siblings (brothers and sisters) in the same terms as buying a product, but the important idea here is that interactions are exchanges. Again, for future positive interactions to occur, the exchange must be fair.

Reciprocity can also refer to the way that your actions influence how people act toward you and vice versa. That is, if you are nice to a person, the person is likely to reciprocate—that is, be nice back to you. If on the other hand, for some reason you act angrily or unkindly toward a friend, your friend is likely to be hurt and behave in the same way toward you. The same is true of the behavior of your friends; if they consistently do things you do not like, the friendship probably will not last very long. As a consequence, to maintain long-term friendships and relationships, positive reinforcement should be used to increase desirable behavior and extinction to decrease undesirable behavior. For instance, everyone likes to be told they look nice, but do you want to reinforce someone by telling her/him how nice he/she looks when wearing a dirty old sweat shirt and torn jeans? What if one of your friends has a tendency to use bad language when you are around? You might not mind if you are alone, but what if you are around your parents or grandparents or other adults who do mind? In this situation, you would probably want to ignore the bad language by walking away and/or doing something else (extinction) until your friend stops. As you can see, the techniques you have learned (reinforcement, extinction, and shaping) can be used in many situations to maintain fair equitable relationships.

One final point needs to be covered concerning the use of behavioral procedures or skills, and that is ethics. Is it unfair or unethical?

Ethics

Is it unethical *deliberately* to change a person's behavior without that person knowing about it? This is a very difficult question to answer. The word deliberately was emphasized because we often change or influence people's behavior by accident—that is, without thinking about or planning our actions. Similarly, we may systematically try to change another person's behavior but not think of it in ethical terms. For instance, a teacher instructing students on how to do long division problems or to write a sentence using a prepositional phrase is systematically trying to change the student's behavior. The people who design television advertisements are also trying to change the viewer's behavior in ways that make it more likely that the viewer will buy the product being advertised. Nonetheless, the question remains, Under what circumstances is an individual obligated to tell the other person of an effort to change that person's behavior? My personal rule of thumb is this: If I am going to be collecting data on the individual's behavior, I tell the person and ask permission. In my interactions with friends and family, I try to reinforce positive responses and extinguish negative ones. I do not ask my friends for permission to reinforce them. But if one of my friends were to come to me and seek my professional help as a psychologist, I would carefully explain what we would do and then make sure my friend understood and agreed before going on. I do essentially the same thing with anyone who consults me professionally or participates in one of the many experiments I conduct.

In short, when one individual is systematically manipulating variables (whether these are medical, economic, or psychological) that can influence another person's life, the first person is ethically obligated to inform the second about the experiment. On the other hand, if you are trying to reduce the friction between your mother and yourself by promptly arriving home at the agreed time and speaking more positively when you and she are not arguing, you are simply trying to improve your life and need not worry about such things as informed consent. The main consideration in using behavior modification procedures to improve your own life is to be fair and honest with people. If you consider the other person's feelings and follow that general rule, it is likely that you will have many warm friendships.

Study Guide

1. You need to be aware of the

    _____ of your behavior on other

    people.

2. Behavior modification skills should be used to the

    _____ of the people you interact

    with as well as yourself.

3. Some "problem students" were taught how to

    _____ their teachers.

4. The reinforcement procedure resulted in the teachers paying more

   _____ to these students. The students and their teachers also got along

   _____.

5. Many people who have interpersonal difficulties do not

   _____ how their behavior affects others.

6. The term _____ is used for a relationship where both people benefit.

7. For relationships to be maintained, they must be

   _____.

8. Interactions can be viewed as psychological

   _____ between two people or groups of people.

9. The important factor in determining whether an exchange is equitable is whether both parties view it as

   _____.

Project Report on a Study to Improve a Friendship

The following report was written by a young woman who found that she was spending too much time fighting with her friend over the friend's critical and negative comments. She decided to change the way she reacted to her friend's critical comments to see if that would help.

Self-Management Project
Julie L.
6th. Period Mr. H.

I conducted this project because I was fighting with my best friend most of the time. Maybe I am too sensitive, but it seemed like every time she said anything it criticized me or some of our other friends. So I would be negative back and we would end up arguing and sometimes yelling real loud. Becaue we had been friends for a long time since 3rd grade I decided to try some behavior [modification] on myself and her.

The self-management project was performed over a period of seven weeks. Baseline$_1$ Treatment$_1$ Baseline$_2$ and Treatment$_2$ data were measured. The behavioral definition stated subject 1 would either leave the room for one minute or if that was not possible ignore subject 2 when she spoke negatively or critical. The results exhibited a decrease in negative and critical comments by subject 2.

Subjects

Both Ss are 14 years of age and are classmates. Subject 1 was imposing the treatment on S2 every time she spoke negatively and/or critical of someone or something.

Method
    Baseline data was collected for two weeks prior to treatment. The treatment condition—S1 would leave the room for one minute or ignore what S2 said was used when S1 thought it was appropriate. S1 was careful to speak with S2 when she was not acting negatively or critical. Therefore, S2 would try and gain attention with negative action but positive conversations. Baseline 2 data was then measured for one week after treatment. To be honest I just forgot to ignore her for a couple of days and when she started being negative, I decided to go ahead for a week to see what would happen. The next week I went back to ignoring her negative comments.

Results and Discussion
    The treatment condition must have been a success for there was a decrease in the negativism of S2. It is not known whether S2 still remains negative when S1 is not with her. This could be a fault in the design. S1 could be a discriminative stimulus for S2 to behave differently. The mean in $Baseline_1$ is 5.64 and in $Baseline_2$ is 4.0 while in Treatment (1) it is 3.2, and Treatment (2), 1.8.

    Although there are a number of important mistakes in this report (she never gives a definition of negative comments), you can get a pretty good idea of what Julie did and how it turned out. Review her report and make a list of the mistakes you think she may have made both in conducting her project and writing the report. After you have completed that, discuss Julie's project in class, including how well it was done and whether you think she acted ethically toward her friend when she changed both her own behavior and that of her friend.

A Behavior Analysis Project: Improving a Friendship

Sarah's program to change her behavior and make friends with Raphael, Jim, and Amy was a behavior modification study. Sarah's goal was to make friends because she had none. The goal of the present experiment is not to make friends but to improve your interactions with a particular friend. We all have friends that we like very much but who nonetheless do things that annoy us and interfere with the friendship. Perhaps they tease us about our large ears, make fun of other friends, or always have to have the final say on what to do or where to go. Such behavior reduces the equity or fairness of the friendship and may well result in your terminating (stopping) the relationship. Friendships frequently end because of arguments over just these kinds of behaviors. Rather than arguing with your friend over the particular behavior that is bothering you, you could try to change that response by changing the way you act.

Method

Subject

You should conduct this study with someone you know and generally like. The person should also be someone you would like to be better friends with if he/she did not have some habit that annoyed you.

Because this is an experiment, it is important that your friend agrees to participate. You should obtain his/her *informed consent* by sitting down with your friend and explaining the basic idea of the experiment. It should be explained that you will be trying to change systematically the way you act when with this person. You should also explain that you will be recording how he/she reacts. Give a general example of how you will behave; for example, instead of arguing when your friend makes a "sarcastic" remark, you will simply ignore it, so that he/she understands what you are trying to do. Be sure to explain carefully how the results of the experiment should help make the two of you better friends. Because it is sometimes hard to explain an experiment without confusing the listener, the class should practice the informed consent procedure. This can be done by having one person play the role of the subject and a second person pretend to be the experimenter. The people can then exchange roles so that each person has experience explaining his/her experiment to another person before trying it with the friend.

Dependent Measures

You will need to define carefully two responses or sets of responses. The first response will be the behavior that bothers you about your friend. For the sake of example, let us say that your friend tends to make too many sarcastic or cruel remarks. To conduct the experiment, a behavioral definition of sarcastic remarks is needed. While everyone "knows" what a sarcastic remark is, a more specific or precise method of identifying one is needed for research. Sarcastic remarks directed at an individual are phrases or comments that ridicule some characteristic of a person's physical features and/or his/her behavior. Statements such as "How ya doin', pig eyes?" "Way to go, graceful," or "You've got the brains of a gnat," are clearly sarcastic. For the purpose of the experiment, you can probably make a list of sarcastic remarks that your friend often uses. The list could then be used as the definition for the experiment. If it is a behavior other than sarcastic remarks that bothers you, the same general procedures can be used to develop a behavioral definition for that response.

The second behavior should be a response that is *incompatible* with the target behavior selected for the experiment. For the example of sarcastic remarks, *positive comments* about your appearance and/or behavior would make a good second response category. The idea here is to select a set of responses that you would like to have your friend make more often and that also make it harder for him/her to engage in the less desirable response. If, instead of sarcastic remarks, you had chosen to target the behavior regarding who decides what the two of you will do, then asking your opinion or ideas for what to do would make a good incompatible response to study. Irrespective of which two sets of responses you decide to work on, they should be carefully defined so that you can accurately record their occurrence.

Recording Procedures

In order to collect data on your friend's behavior, you will need a very simple recording system. Though you will have told your friend already that you will be recording how he/she reacts to you, it would be awkward to be writing everything down as you talk or do other things together. Probably the simplest procedure to use is to carry a small notebook. *Every morning*, write the day's date on the top of a new page, and then also write the definitions of the behaviors that you are observing. This will help you remember exactly what behaviors you are concerned with so that you will automatically recognize them. During the day, after you have interacted with your friend and you are alone, simply record the time and how many times each behavior occurred. In the evening you should review your notes to make sure you have recorded each occurrence of the behaviors.

You have used *extinction* in previous experiments. For this experiment, the extinction procedure will consist of ignoring (doing nothing) in response to a sarcastic remark and breaking eye contact for a brief period of time. When we speak to another person, we usually look at the person. This attention often functions as a form of positive reinforcement. During the extinction procedure, when the subject begins to make a sarcastic remark, simply look away, look at the desk, the wall, over your friend's shoulder, etc. until the statement is over and he/she is talking about something else. Then you can again look at the person and make eye contact. Do not make any comment or argue in any way with your friend about the sarcastic remark, simply ignore it. You should continue the conversation as if nothing had happened.

You will *reinforce* positive comments by attending when such comments are made. Suppose the subject compliments you on your test grade, you should follow that response with an appropriate positive comment about the subject, such as, I am sure you will do well on the math test today, or that's really nice of you to say so, or a simple expression of interest, such as mmhm, or even a smile and good eye contact. All of these consequences can function as positive reinforcers. If you use a mix of them, it is likely that some of them will serve as positive reinforcers for your friend.

You should begin the experiment by collecting a *baseline record* of how often your friend makes sarcastic remarks and positive comments to you before anything is done. The baseline should consist of 1 week of recording. You will record the occurrence of the two behaviors anytime you are interacting with your friend.

After collecting the baseline data, the *experimental condition* will be instituted the next day. Again, you will record data whenever you two interact, but now you will attend to and show interest when your friend makes positive comments and break eye contact and generally ignore your friend when he/she makes sarcastic remarks. Implement the experimental condition for 2 weeks.

Data Analysis

To analyze the results of your experiment, make two graphs—one for positive comments and one for sarcastic remarks. Compare baseline levels of each response to the levels found in the experimental condition. Theoretically, if everything worked properly, the frequency of positive comments should have increased during the experimental condition and the frequency of sarcastic remarks should have decreased in comparison to the baseline. Remember, when analyzing your data, you are comparing the frequencies of responses found in the *experimental condition* to those observed during the baseline and not to each other.

UNIT 22

Contracting and Negotiating

A contract is a formal or informal agreement between two or more persons that specifies what each party should do and what the consequences will be of those actions. Family interactions are typically centered around unwritten or unstated contracts. Usually, these contracts develop over time and are based on the needs and expectations of the people involved. However, this form of contract is not very reliable. Very often, as a matter of fact, this unwritten contract leads to misunderstandings and a breakdown in family communication. This breakdown is usually started because parents, as their children get older, have difficulty giving them age-appropriate responsibility. At the same time, children are sometimes lacking in the skills necessary to talk to their parents and express their needs.

Psychologists who work with families in which there are communication problems between parents and their children have developed some procedures that lead to better communication. These procedures can also help improve communication in families that are only having small problems. The primary method used is a contract, which specifies who is to do what for whom under what circumstances. In other words, contracting allows for compromise so that all members of the family can maximize positive reinforcement and minimize any losses the contract may call for. The skill that is of utmost importance in contracting is negotiation.

The role of negotiation in developing contracts among family members first requires that any discussion concerning the contract be *open, honest*, and *free from pressure* on all sides. Second, the terms of the contract should be stated simply and clearly in *writing*, with all aspects completely specified. Third, *reinforcers* and *consequences* for complying or not complying with the contract should be specified for all persons involved. The final rule in establishing contracts is to be sure that those persons involved are successful in fulfilling the terms of the contract. To make sure this happens, all contracted behavior should be in the person's behavioral repertoire. That is, the contract should only call for the person to do things he/she has done in the past. Very often, when families are drawing up contracts they expect too much at one time. For instance, parents may expect their teenager to improve his/her school grades to all A's at one time. This, of course, may be too much to expect, so a more appropriate contract would be to improve a grade in one class at a time. Once the grade in that class reaches the criteria specified in the contract, then another class may be added.

When the actual aspects of a contract are negotiated, it is, of course, desirable for all persons involved to be present. Usually, it is helpful if special attention is taken as to how a person presents her/himself physically. Being neatly dressed with your hair combed can help a lot when negotiating with adults. Now consider this example of how a contracting situation might work: The topic will be the hour at which a 13-year-old boy, Jason, can stay out on weekdays and weekend nights. The current situation that is causing problems is that the parents want Jason home at 8:00 P.M. on week nights, and 10:00 P.M. on weekend nights. Jason states that he feels 9:00 on week nights and 12:00 on weekends would be more appropriate because these are the times that most of his friends must be home. His parents think that this is much too late and that it won't allow him enough time to complete his homework and household chores. Also, his parents are concerned about where Jason would be this late at night. Jason and his parents then agree that he is to be home at 11:30 on weekend nights. But his parents aren't satisfied because this doesn't solve the problems with homework and household chores. Jason's parents then offer to extend the curfew on week nights to 9:00 P.M. if he agrees to come home directly after school and complete both his homework and his household chores to his parents' satisfaction. After a bit more discussion, Jason and his parents agree to the 9:00 curfew. Jason then offers to call home at 10:30 and 11:30 P.M. on weekend nights and tell his parents where he is. The parents agree that he can stay out until 12:00 midnight if his homework is done, he has completed his household chores, and he remembers to call.

The example of negotiating a contract presented here appears very simple. Not all situations are simple, however; sometimes it is very difficult to reach an agreement that is to everyone's advantage and minimizes any individual losses. The most *important* thing to remember in *contracting* is *to control your temper*; nothing is gained for either side by yelling at each other. Only those topics under discussion should be talked about. It doesn't usually do much good to talk about something that happened 2 or 3 weeks ago, even if it is related to the problem. You should listen carefully and ask questions if you are unaware or unsure of what's being said. Be specific in identifying rewards for yourself and others in your contract proposals. Finally, establish priorities for what should be discussed first, second, and third.

Once the negotiating is completed, you must write the contract. Each person involved should read the written contract and check to see that all aspects are completely specified. When everyone has read and agreed to what is written, all the individuals involved should sign the contract. From the time it is signed until it is no longer relevant or it is renegotiated, every attempt should be made to help it work.

A very important part of good communication is understanding the other person's point of view or position. Although adolescents often feel that their parents don't understand them, parents frequently feel the same way about adolescents. To give you a view from the parents' side of the fence, the following pieces from The Associated Press and *The New York Times* are reprinted here. It is hoped that this information will help you understand how your parents sometimes feel.

Mother strikes; children yield[14]

Associated Press—Vader, Wash.—Gina Smith, a mother who went on strike two weeks ago until her three kids agreed to do more around the house, was back in the kitchen Monday and her children were "bending over backward" to help.

But Smith, 37, said she was formally still on strike because she's had trouble getting her three children together to sign a formal contract outlining their duties around the house.

"My son (Shawn, 16) has ball practice every day after school and the older daughter, Tracee, has swing choir and choir practice. I may have to get them in shifts," she said.

She said she hopes the document will be signed before a notary public by Friday.

Smith, a full-time waitress, went on strike after losing patience with her children, who were critical of her for not doing enough around the house. She vowed not to cook, clean or chauffeur for them, and suspended their $6 weekly allowance.

At first, the youngsters called her "stupid" and were embarrassed by the publicity the strike drew. They lived on cereal, macaroni and cheese, nachos and pizza.

14. Reprinted by permission of The Associated Press.

But then they started pitching in.

"They've been helping each other with their meals and laundry. . . . They fold each other's clothing," Smith said. "Before, they'd just take a pair of socks and throw the rest on the couch. It would sit there a month if I didn't fold it."

"We'll do things now instead of sitting around and saying we'll do the work later," said Kimberly, 13.

"I know now that she puts forth a lot of effort to be a good mom," said Tracee, 16. "She wanted us to see how much she really did."

The Battle Field[15]

New York Times—New York—The day finally came when Roberta Schoenfield could no longer bear to argue with her 13-year-old son, Eric, about the unmade bed in his room and the clutter on the floor.

"I decided that I could pour no more emotional energy into it," Mrs. Schoenfield, the mother of three boys, said, "so I told Eric that I would not enter his room or bother him about it until he began to keep it neat himself on an ongoing basis. In return I told him I would not do his laundry."

So for three months Eric has been washing his clothes and sheets and ironing his shirts, and he is perfectly content with the arrangement.

Their solution may be unusual, but their problem—the adolescent's "messy" room—is virtually universal. And it can be baffling.

"Parents view messiness as a sign of what will continue for the rest of the child's life, and they take it as a personal slap in the face," said Dr. Ralph I. Lopez, director of the division of adolescent medicine at the New York Hospital–Cornell Medical Center.

One mother described the sensation she felt on entering her children's rooms as that of "a knife going into my stomach." Another said, "It tears my insides out, and all I want to do is lash out at them."

To Lopez the issue reflects in some measure the division of rights in a family. "It is really a question of who owns the child's room," he said. "It is the children's idea that 'if this is my room, why can't I keep it the way I want?' versus the parents' contention that 'this is our home so you must abide by our regulations.'"

Jack Amiel, who is almost 15, reflected that difficult balance when he said: "I don't resent it when my mom gets crazy about it. It's my room, and I know I should keep it clean." He paused. "But sometimes I think it is my room and I have the right to keep clutter. Maybe parents have too much power."

Parents use that power—or choose not to use it—in a variety of ways, from shouting to silence. Most clearly consider the issue more a nuisance than divisive matter.

Sallie Bloom of Rye Brook, N.Y., is not happy about the way her daughters, Karen, 13, and Judy, 11, keep their rooms. "Their drawers are open, discarded clothes are on the floor, books and papers on the dressers and night tables, beds are never made," she said. "In the morning they may put on entire outfits and remove them because they don't like the look. They put those clothes in the laundry rather than fold them."

How does Mrs. Bloom, office manager for a computer consulting concern and a caterer, cope? "I have tried everything from screaming to getting Karen up at 2 A.M. on weekends to clean her room," she said. Still, she maintains her perspective. "Both my children are bright, friendly and loving," she said. "Karen cleans the kitchen every night—92 percent as well as I would—and Judy walks the dog."

Nancy Amiel, vice president of a public-relations company in New York City, who describes herself as compulsively neat, said she did not shout at her children. "I suggest, and when I can't get in the door because it is blocked by ski equipment, I order them to clean up their rooms," she said. "But I also feel those rooms are their private turf, so often I just close the door."

Her husband, Joseph, a novelist, is even more philosophical: "Messiness has an entirely different meaning to them. To us it connotes appearance and a sense of order. To them it is simply irrelevant."

Andrea Amiel, 18, agreed, saying: "There are so many more important things to worry about—doing well in school, getting into college—that room cleaning just moves into the background."

Susan Picard, a psychologist and the mother of sons aged 20 and 17 and a daughter, 12, takes a relaxed position. "Those are their rooms and their business," she said, "but once a week they must clean up because it's our home. Theoretically they must make their beds, but I've given up on that because I prefer that they rebel that way rather than do other things. If a child has a good character, is happy, healthy, doing well at school and has friends, then this is hardly something to worry about."

For those who do worry, there is hope, as demonstrated by the case of Nancy Brown and her daughter. Mrs. Brown, an interior decorator who has three children, Margaret, 24, Peter, 20, and Nicholas, 14, said: "The only time they were reasonably neat was when there was someone to pick up after them, myself or a maid. My older son once put dirty dishes in his bed rather than wash them."

Today, Margaret, a production manager for a magazine, has her own apartment, and therein lies the happy ending. "I certainly used to be messy," she said. "It was easier to go along with the hippie mode of thinking, the rebelliousness of it. But now I have my own apartment, and I'm proud of it, so it's very neat."

Study Guide

1. A breakdown in family communication is usually started because

   _____ have difficulty giving their

   children age-appropriate _____.

2. _____ is a method used to develop better communication in the family.

3. The skill that is of the utmost importance in contracting is called

   _____.

4. All discussions concerning contracts should be

   _____,

   _____, and

   _____ on both sides.

5. All contracts should be _____,
   with all aspects stated simply and clearly.

6. The most important rule in establishing contracts is to be sure that

   those involved meet with _____.

7. Only those _____ under dicus-
   sion should be discussed.

8. All persons involved in the contracting situation should be able to

   maximize their _____ and mini-

   mize any _____.

9. Being specific in _____ rewards
   for yourself and others is a primary aspect of a contract.

Relaxation and Biofeedback[16]

Relaxation and biofeedback skills training are two ways to learn greater control over an important problem: tension. Many people choose to smoke cigarettes, take drugs, drink alcohol, or overeat because they say these behaviors help them to relax. Some people complain about feeling "nervous" or "stressed out" or "anxious" in many everyday situations, such as just before a test, in difficult math or science classes, or when asking a friend or an attractive person out on a date. Other people feel "tense" or "uptight" when talking to parents or teachers or when their behavior has led to troublesome consequences. Relaxation and biofeedback are procedures that can help to reduce tension and anxiety in everyday situations.

The following section is a paraphrase of an experiment done by Robin, Schneider, and Dolnick[17] to help overly aggressive children. The study illustrates (1) how tension can be involved in problem behaviors such as aggression and acting out, and (2) how learning to relax helps reduce the frequency of those behaviors.

Report on a Relaxation Procedure for Emotionally Disturbed Children

The "Turtle Technique" is a self-control procedure that was used to help elementary school kids who were so tense that they would become aggressive in their classroom. They were in a special classroom for

16. The first draft of this unit was written by Barbara Wood.

17. See A. Robin, M. Schneider, & M. Dolnick (1976). The Turtle Technique: An extended case study of self-control in the classroom. *Psychology in the Schools, 13,* 94–101.

emotionally disturbed children because they had many problems, hit other children, and were doing very poorly in school. The psychologists who created this relaxation technique to help the young children hypothesized that if they could teach the children to relax, then the children would probably hit other children less frequently during stressful school situations.

They thought that it was also important to make learning fun. What could be a better way to teach kids to relax than to tell them a story? So they began with this story:

> . . . Little Turtle was a handsome young turtle who was very upset about going to school. He always got in trouble at school because he got into fights. Other kids would tease, bump, or hit him: He would get very angry and start big fights. The teacher would have to punish him. Then one day he met the big old tortoise, who told him that his shell was the secret answer to all his problems. The tortoise told Little Turtle to withdraw into his shell when he felt angry and rest until he was no longer angry. So he tried it the next day, and it worked. The teacher now smiled at him and he no longer got into big fights.

The children said they liked the story so much that they wanted to learn how to "do a turtle." "Doing a turtle" was another name for doing a relaxation exercise. Just as a turtle withdraws into his or her shell when there is trouble, the children were taught to relax rather than to fight.

The psychologists used a technique called *progressive muscle relaxation* to teach the children and their teacher to "do a turtle." The benefit of progressive muscle relaxation is that it helps people to notice and let go of the tension in their muscles. Muscle tension is associated with what many people call "nervousness," "anxiety," "being stressed out," "uptight," or "tense." The target behavior of progressive muscle relaxation, or the "turtle technique," is being able to relax the muscles of the body during stressful life situations. In relaxation, you must be able to *discriminate* when you are tensing your muscles and to learn how to let go of the muscle tension in each part of the body to relax.

Stress has become a popular term. It means that the environment is putting a demand on the person to change or to adjust to some new demand. Any change in the environment that requires a change in the person's behavior can be seen as a stressful situation.

For the children who learned the "turtle technique," stressful situations in the environment included working on a difficult math problem that made the children feel angry or frustrated with themselves or being taunted to fight by a kid who was name calling or punching. These situations were considered stressful because, by definition, stress is re-lated to a demand or pressure from the environment to change. The students were being pressured to complete a difficult math problem or to handle a possible fight. These were stressful situations.

In these stressful situations, the teacher or another student who saw what was happening was taught to call out "turtle" or "do a turtle." The child who was tensing his/her muscles in frustration was taught to imagine that he/she was a turtle withdrawing into the shell, by pulling his/her arms close to the body, putting the head down on the desk, and closing the eyes. Thus, the child learned the skill of how to first tense and then relax each muscle in the body. By learning certain exercises (similar to exercises in gym class), the children learned to notice or *discriminate* between the feeling of tension followed by the feeling of relaxation in each muscle of the body.

All of the children in the class practiced progressive muscle relaxa-tion and the "turtle response" *every day*. They were rewarded for practic-ing the skill every day, and after a few weeks, the children had learned the skill. Usually, when the teacher or another student called a "turtle," the child who was tensing his/her muscle did the "turtle response" and then did a progressive muscle relaxation exercise.

During the experiment, the psychologists collected data during a 2-week *baseline*. They measured the number of aggressive behaviors shown by the entire group in a week. "Aggressive behavior" was *operationally defined* as a behavior in which a child made a forceful movement directed at either another person or an object, including hitting, throwing objects, kicking, grabbing, tearing up his/her or another's materials, and so on. The group of children in the class showed a weekly mean (average) number of aggressive behaviors equal to 20 during the *baseline condition*. By the end of the *treatment condition*, the group showed a weekly mean of 12 aggressive behaviors. The children decreased the number of aggres-sive behaviors by 41% by doing the turtle technique.

Reducing the frequency of aggressive behavior is just one example of how relaxation skills have helped people to control their own behavior. I am sure we have all noticed that if we are tired or tense, we are more likely to become upset or snap at others when small things go wrong. When we are irritable, trivial things make us mad that would ordinarily be ignored. Recognizing that I am acting unreasonable does not help, but learning simple relaxation skills can. Fortunately, you don't have to be a turtle to use these techniques.

Like any new skill, *practice* is very important. To start, you will need to choose a comfortable, quiet spot to lie down or rest your head on the back of a chair or on your desk. Next, the teacher or a student with a calm, quiet tone of voice will be chosen to read the instructions from the instructors' guide.[18]

The basic steps are as follows:

1. Get comfortable and close your eyes.
2. Now breathe deeply.
3. Breathe in and breathe out slowly and deeply.
4. Think of your diaphragm as a balloon. Your diaphragm is located just below your stomach. As you breathe in and out, think of moving your diaphragm up and down as if blowing up a balloon each time you breathe in deeply and slowly breathe out.
5. Once you've got the breathing technique down, rest in your comfortable position and continue breathing deeply, blowing up the balloon as you breathe in, then slowly letting all the air out.

It also can be very relaxing to picture something special in your mind as you breathe in and breathe out and as you listen to the suggestions for relaxing each muscle in your body. Some students enjoy imagining a beautiful scene such as the ocean and the beach. They imagine seeing the beautiful colors of the water and sky, the sun glistening on the water, and they can feel the warmth of sun on their skin; they hear the seagulls flying and taste the saltiness of the sea on their lips in their imagination. Relaxation skills are most effective when a student chooses his/her own special image for relaxation. You can also say things to yourself such as "I feel warm and relaxed," "Stay cool," "Relax," or "I'm in control of relaxation." Again, the skill will be most helpful if you choose a special pleasant thought or word just for you.

Now that you are choosing to get comfortable, to breathe deeply, and perhaps to imagine a relaxing scene or pleasant word or thought, let's begin. (The instructor or student now reads the progressive, muscle relaxation suggestions.)

After the exercise, make out a record of your practice times. You can do this by rating how relaxed you felt from 1 to 10, where 1 means extremely tense and 10 means completely relaxed. Practice the skill each day for 15 to 20 minutes and record your tension level based on the 1 to 10 point scale. You should keep your record in a notebook and review it periodically to see if you're making progress.

Because most people find the physical feelings of relaxation very pleasant or rewarding, as you improve your efforts at relaxation, you

---

18. A tape recording of these instructions can be used instead of having someone read the instructions each time.

should be positively reinforced by those feelings of increased relaxation. Your *self-monitoring* of relaxation will make it easier to see your progress and will encourage you to continue trying.

Biofeedback is another procedure that can be used, along with progressive muscle relaxation to help people get better control over tension. The term *biofeedback* is a contraction of biological feedback. You are already familiar with the term feedback. That is what teachers do when they give you grades. One of the problems with grades as feedback is that they are delayed—they are "fed back" too long after the relevant responses. The psychologist, Neal Miller, discovered that by providing *immediate* feedback on a biological response, such as muscle contraction or tension, and constriction or dilation of the blood vessels, and so forth, you can actually teach organisms to control these ANS responses. In a classic study, Miller and his associates provided rats with tones indicating whether their blood vessels were constricting or dilating. Using this feedback, the rats learned to dilate the blood vessels of one ear *while* constricting the vessels in the other ear! Many psychologists then automatically assumed that if rats could do it, people could learn to control important ANS responses as well. Nevertheless, it took considerably more research before effective biofeedback procedures were developed for humans.

Biofeedback training helps people to objectively measure their level of muscle tension. By giving immediate feedback as to whether their tension level increases or decreases, biofeedback allows them to *discriminate* better between the feeling of tension or relaxation in their muscles. The electromyograph (EMG) is an electronic self-monitoring device that measures the level of tension in the muscles. To measure tension, surface electrodes are attacked to the skin on the forehead, neck, or arm. The EMG takes information obtained by the surface electrodes and electronically changes the information into feedback that can be understood. A sound that gets louder or softer depending on how tense or relaxed a person gets is one kind of biofeedback. Hearing the sound get louder helps the person to discriminate that he or she is becoming more tense.

Inside of the EMG is an amplifier; like those used in stereo equipment. The amplifier of a radio or stereo changes the sound waves broadcasted from radio stations into the music we hear. The EMG works the same way when it changes electronic information from the electrons on the surface of the skin or from the muscles right below the skin into the tones we hear.

If you can borrow an EMG, some simple exercises may help you to understand better how the electromyogram works and how you can learn to better control your own muscle tension. For the exercise you will need the following:

1. Graph paper
2. An EMG
3. A student to record data
4. A student volunteer to get "hooked up" to the EMG
5. A student to keep track of the time intervals
6. A stopwatch

During the first part of this exercise, experiment with the biofeed-back equipment and recording data, to observe your levels of muscle tension under different conditions. For example, for 15 seconds one student could first tense his/her muscles tightly. The recorder might read 40 microvolts on the EMG display and record it. For the next 15 seconds, the student would relax and breathe deeply. The recorder might read 20 microvolts. Also the students would have heard the biofeedback sound get softer and softer as the student relaxed. Suppose a baseline reading of 30 microvolts had been taken for 30 seconds prior to begin-ning the experimental procedure. Then, during the second part of the activity, the person should try to relax so deeply that the sound goes off completely. Once the students have practiced progressive muscle relaxa-tion, they should be able to turn off the sound completely. Keep a record of the number of microvolts read during several 15-minute practice sessions over a week, to see if you can control the tension in your muscles. This activity could be done in small groups. Perhaps the instruc-tor could offer a reward to the small group that has shown the most practice, as measured by the lowest number of microvolts recorded in 1 week.

Study Guide

1. Progressive relaxation is a procedure that can reduce

   _____ and

   _____ .

2. _____ can be associated with undesirable behaviors such as aggression, emotional outbursts, and so on.

3. What does it mean to do a turtle?

_____

4. When the children were in a

_____ situation, they were sup-

posed to do a turtle.

5. Sometimes it helps to _____ a

pleasant scene in the relaxation procedure.

6. Biofeedback is a method of controlling some

_____

_____

_____ responses.

7. Biofeedback works by providing

_____ changes in a tone when

there is a change in the response.

8. The _____ is used to measure

muscle tension.

UNIT 24

Self-Management

In the previous units, we have discussed applying the procedures of reinforcement, and extinction to improve relations with friends, teachers, and family. Now we are going to learn how to use self-control or self-management to influence your own behavior by these same procedures. Self-management should ideally represent an approach to life in which an individual accepts responsibility for his/her own behavior. If a behavior is unacceptable to you, then you should take steps to produce a more desirable behavior.

The steps in a self-management program are the same as the steps in any behavior change program. The first step is to establish a goal—that is, decide which behavior you would like to change. Then clearly, in writing, identify and define the target behavior. Next, you should measure the target response recording either frequency (if the behavior is discrete) or duration (if it is continuous). This preliminary period of measurement will establish a baseline condition in which you can determine the natural occurrence of the behavior. In the intervention plan to alter the behavior, remember that if you want to increase the frequency, use reinforcement; to decrease the frequency, use either response cost or extinction. Finally, continue monitoring the behavior until you have reached your goal.

Basic to the use of self-management techniques is the ability to analyze your own behavior. Often, our own behavior doesn't seem to make sense until we stop to analyze it in terms of the consequences for those responses. For instance, we may repeatedly behave in ways that we really don't like and would like to stop, but because we don't understand why we are doing those things in the first place, we are unable to stop and only become more frustrated. Frequently, we find that there are some small immediate reinforcers that support the behavior and make it difficult to quit. To take a concrete example, everyone knows that smoking is bad for you, yet many people who would like to quit find it almost impossible to do so. Why is that? Even though smoking may lead to lung cancer, emphysema, heart disease, loss of teeth through gum disease, and the like, these consequences are *delayed*. That is, you don't immediately have a small heart attack each time you light a cigarette and inhale. Rather, there are small but immediate positive reinforcers for smoking. When the smoker inhales, immediately the smoker tastes the tobacco, feels the nicotine (drug) start to circulate in the body, and may feel more relaxed. The smoker may receive social approval from friends. Finally, if the smoker is not yet an adult, he/she may feel more adult or mature when smoking. In short, a whole variety of potential positive reinforcers occur immediately while smoking. Research has shown that even small immediate consequences have very powerful effects on behavior even though there may be important delayed detrimental (bad) consequences for the response, as in the case of smoking. So if someone wishes to stop smoking, the person needs to be able to identify the immediate positive consequences and eliminate them.

We discuss smoking in greater detail later in the manual, so let us now consider another example. Suppose that you have gotten into the habit of teasing your sister. You would like to stop because you would like to get along better with her; and there are other obvious delayed aversive consequences for continuously teasing your sister: She is less likely to help you when you need help; you are often punished by your parents for teasing her; and occasionally she gets mad enough to hit you or break something of yours. With all those bad things that happen when you tease her, why do you still do it? Somehow, no matter how hard you try, you can't resist the opportunity to make fun of her, tease her, and so on. What is going on here?

To answer that question, we have to ask what happens immediately when you tease her? Does she get embarrassed, angry, cry? As strange as it may seem, your sister's reactions may be positive reinforcers for your teasing. You must have known someone at school who seemed to go out of his/her way to bother the teacher. Getting the teacher's goat (making him/her mad) was probably a positive reinforcer for that person. Similarly, you may be rewarded by your sister's anger. If that is the case, what can you do about it?

First, you need to find out more about your teasing behavior. Start by taking a baseline and record the situations when you tease your sister. You need to know whether you tease her when you are alone or when other people are there (e.g., are your parents there?). Does she usually do something to you first? Do you usually tease her at home or at school or maybe even at a friend's house? In short, the more information you can get about your teasing behavior, the better chance you have of changing it.

For instance, let's say that your sister gets better grades in school than you do and you discover that you usually start teasing her when she is bragging about schoolwork or your parents are praising her for something she did in school. Now that you know when you are likely to tease her, you can do something about it. Maybe when your parents are praising her you might say something nice also. When you are nice to someone, the person is usually nice back; when you praise someone, the person usually tries to say something good about you. There is also a good chance that your parents will notice the difference and try to talk about something you have done well that day. When you are alone with your sister, you might try to ignore (extinguish) her bragging and pay attention to (reinforce) her when she is talking about something that is of interest to you. Soon, you and she will talk to one another without getting into a fight and perhaps you might even get to be friends. But remember that it is important to record what you do and how people react. The first things you try might not work, but if you keep records it will be easier for you to think of new things to try. Also, it is important to keep good records so you will know how well your program is working.

You should have noticed that in this hypothetical example, you not only changed your own behavior, but also the behavior of your sister and your parents. Such an outcome is not uncommon, in fact, anytime you change some social behavior—either your own or somebody else's—there will be a mutual change in your own or that person's behavior. Remember the case of Sarah—she decided to change the behavior of some of her classmates, but the only way she could accomplish this task was to change her own behavior.

Sarah's goal was to make friends with three of the students in her class—Jim, Amy, and Raphael. Her target for the first 3 weeks was to get one or more of them to say nice things to her. But first she monitored or measured the baseline rate by noting on a small card she carried around the number of bad and good things that were said to her by these three people. Next, she decided that she would (1) reinforce any nice comments by helping or talking to them, and (2) extinguish any negative comments by turning her back or walking away from them. The results were that these three people started making more positive comments to Sarah and being more friendly in general. Of course, not only did Jim, Amy, and Raphael change their behavior, but Sarah also changed, in that she was friendlier and more fun to be around.

Not all self-management projects involve your social behavior or somebody else's. Let's say, for example, that you bite your fingernails, and, as a result, your hands are red, pretty well beat up, and—on occasion—hurt. The first step has been done—we have identified the target response—

stopping fingernail biting. Now, because you are interested in decreasing the number of *times* you bite your nails, what method of measurement should you use? Frequency. It is important when you begin monitoring the behavior that you note not only how many times you bite your fingernails, but also when you do it. Can you think of why this would be important? Because you can now identify certain places and times during the day when you are biting your nails the most. In altering the behavior, you may have to think about other things you can do physically to prevent nail biting. If you have noticed that you bite your nails, for instance, when talking to members of the opposite sex, you can (1) begin to place your hands behind your back or in your pockets or (2) do something else with them in this situation. Or, if you bite your nails a lot when you are studying, you can practice keeping your hands pressed down firmly on the top of your desk. In some situations, like nail biting, you may want to tell some of your friends or family that if they can catch you biting your nails that you must pay them a nickel or a dime.

Behavioral procedures can be used in a wide variety of ways to increase your ability to control your behavior. The next units concern the use of these procedures in a relaxation project and a weight-control program. After you read and discuss these units, you will be asked to design and conduct your own self-management experiment. So in reviewing this unit and the next ones, you should be thinking about ways you can use self-management techniques to solve a personal difficulty.

Study Guide

1. Self-management is a method of using behavioral procedures to

   _____ your own behavior.

2. Basic to self-management is

   _____ your own behavior.

3. In analysis, the objective is to find the

   _____ that are affecting your behavior.

4. In self-control problems, there are usually small

   _____ reinforcers that control the behavior while there are major

_____ consequences associated
with it.

5. How is smoking a self-control problem?

_____

6. The first step in finding out why you do something such as teasing
   your sister is collect a _____.

7. To change a behavior, you need to know not only the consequences of
   that behavior, but also the _____
   in which you are likely to engage in that behavior.

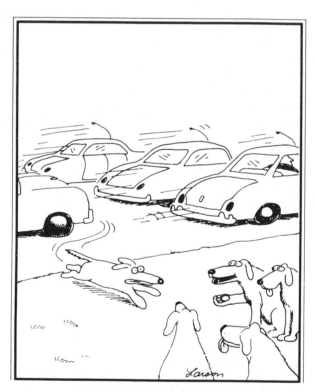

"All right! Rusty's in the club!"

Peer reinforcement often plays an important role in self-control problems. *The Far
Side* cartoon reprinted by permission of Chronicle Features, San Francisco.

UNIT 25

Fear of Public Speaking: Report of a Student's Self-Management Project

Last year I was asked to run for a student body office. At first I agreed but the thought of giving a campaign speech in front of the student body made me more and more nervous. So finally I said no, I really did not want to. It was all very embarrassing. This year I was asked again and decided with some encouragement from my friends to try. Instead of risking making a fool of myself in the speech in front of everybody, I made giving the speech my self-management project.

Obviously, my main fear was making a fool of myself and looking like an idiot. Thinking about everybody looking at me and me making a mistake and everybody laughing at me really made me worried.

Method
Behavioral Definition: Fear of Public Speaking

There seemed to be two things that bothered me. First the idea of being in front of all of the other students with them looking at me, and second the fear of making a stupid mistake in my speech.

I certainly did not take a baseline. Last year all I had to do was think about it and it was enough to make me chicken out.

Program

After thinking about the problem, the first thing I did was get a book on public speaking and read it. There were a lot of good ideas but the first step was to write a good speech. So I wrote the whole thing out. Then I asked some friends and my mother to read it. They made some suggestions and some sarcastic remarks (not my mother). I made some changes and then I was confident that at least the talk wasn't stupid. Next I made note cards on big cards with big type so they would be easy to read and I underlined the main points so that I wouldn't get confused. Next I practiced giving the talk in front of a mirror so I could look up every now and then and practice smiling.

When I had learned my talk, I asked some friends to help me by listening to me give my speech. We met after school in one of the classrooms. We did everything like it was the real thing. Someone introduced me as the candidate for student body treasurer, and I got up and came to the front of the room. I went through the whole thing trying to smile and make eye contact changing the sound of my voice some and all the other techniques in the book. Next the self-management class teacher let me give my speech to the class (a closer approximation to talking in front of everybody). Again, I was introduced and I tried to imagine I was getting up in front of the student body and staying relaxed and smiling. At the front of the room I went through the whole routine of smiling, relaxing and not starting until my breathing was even. That went very well so I was very confident. The last thing I did, believe it or not, was to go to the gym after school and practice going up to the front arranging my notes, relaxing and looking out at all the students I imagined being out there.

The afternoon of the speeches I was a little nervous but I knew I was prepared. So I concentrated on keeping my breathing relaxed and smiling. I didn't look at my speech because I knew it and when it was my turn I just walked up there, relaxed and then looked at everybody and smiled.

Everything went smooth as silk and I got lots of congratulations from everybody afterwards. Unfortunately, a good speech wasn't quite enough and I lost by 5 votes. But it doesn't matter too much because being congratulated by people was fun and actually giving the speech was OK, in fact, it turned out that I liked having all those people listening to me. So I will probably run for the student senate from my home room next fall or something like that.

This project was based on both the self-management procedures we have discussed and common sense. The student, George, analyzed his problem and then developed a plan. First, he learned about public speaking and about writing a good speech. Next, he took care of the nervousness (anxiety) that had stopped him in the past by using a shaping procedure in which he went through successive approximations to giving the talk. Finally, he tried to make the whole thing positive by smiling a lot and keeping his breathing smooth and relaxed.

Overall, the project reflects the sort of planning, preparation and practice that can help a person overcome his/her fears about a stimulus or a situation.

UNIT 26

Weight Control: Report of a Student's Self-Management Project

The following report was written by a girl, Tricia, who used a self-management program to change her eating habits and lose weight. As you read this report, you should outline the major points of what she did. An important feature of this study was Tricia's analysis of her baseline data. She discovered that she was more likely to eat fattening snacks on those days when she had something sweet for breakfast. This turned out to be a key behavior; when she stopped eating sweets for breakfast, it was much easier to control her eating the rest of the day. Remember, a major reason for collecting a baseline on the problem response is to discover just this sort of information.

Final report

The target behavior I chose to change for my self-management project was my snacking. I defined snacking as "the consumption of food or beverage at any time of the day with the exception of breakfast, lunch, and dinner."

After I selected my target behavior, I then recorded my snacking behavior for fourteen days—writing down the date, time and place the snacking took place, as well as what the snack was. This information became my baseline data.

As I analyzed my baseline data, I discovered several patterns in my snacking. I noticed that I tended to have a snack as soon as I walked in the door after school. I also found myself consuming another snack at approximately 8:00 P.M. Many times as I watched T.V., I felt compelled to snack even though I was not hungry. I also tended to snack if I knew there was something to eat in the house. An interesting factor I had not previously noticed was that I tended to snack more frequently during the day if I ate someting sweet for breakfast.

After analyzing my baseline, I proposed to alter my snacking behavior in three ways. First, I removed all the prepared snacks from home and asked my mother not to buy any more. Secondly, I decided to buy some magazines to read for a couple of hours each day after school instead of watching T.V. My third step was to eat a breakfast each day that did not include sweet foods.

After I drew up my proposal, I recorded my snacking behavior for another 14 days abiding by the rules. My snacking changed dramatically! I managed to cut my snacking rate in half. Also the snacks that I did consume were more nutritious, and without all that extra sugar, I did not feel compelled to eat as much over all.

Another interesting factor I discovered was that I was not also tempted to snack when high calory prepared snacks were not easily available. When I knew this stuff was around, psychologically I justified my eating to myself by saying I couldn't let it go to waste.

As far as buying magazines were concerned, this proposal was not quite as successful. Magazines are very expensive, and my budget did not

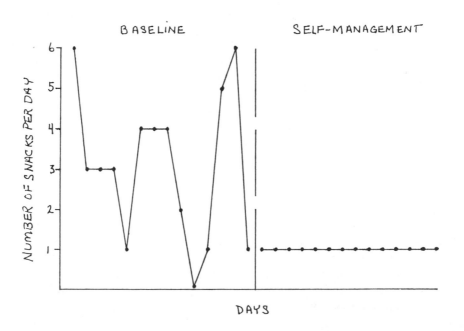

allow me to buy very many. I found myself still watching T.V., but because the prepared snacks were not available I did not snack too much.

Overall, I believe that my project was successful, and I will be rewarded with a thinner and healthier body in the future. I have finally reached terms with myself because I now realize that I can live without the extra snacking, and I am feeling much better about myself both physically and mentally.

You should have noticed that all the things Tricia did to change her snacking involved antecedent (things present before she snacked) stimulus control factors. The two main changes were not eating sweets at breakfast and removing the prepared snacks at home. Eliminating the snack foods changed the situation so that she no longer had to resist the temptation to snack. Eliminating a stimulus in advance is much easier to do than resisting the temptation later on.

UNIT 27

Impatience:
Report of a Student's
Self-Management Project

The self-management project you just read dealt with eating behavior and weight control. While weight control is a difficult problem, actual eating behavior is relatively easy to define and measure. This self-management report concerns a student's effort to understand and control her difficulties with impatience.

Behavioral Definition: Finding it hard to wait for people when I'm ready to go.

1. Start pacing around—can't sit still.
2. Gradually get irritable.
3. Start yelling out "let's go!"
4. Pushing people along—(not physical) getting them to get moving.

Baseline Data: Monitoring what caused my impatient behavior, at what particular times.

1. Waiting for someone after school with two other friends. We were going bowling. Person still not showing up. At first, couldn't sit still and started pacing around, asked friends where he could be and tried calling on phone to see if he had even left yet. I found myself, getting really irritable, I kept looking at the clock every 30 seconds, and by the time he finally showed up I was more mad then anything else.

2. Trying to call home but the line is busy. Knowing it's most likely my little sister. I started dialing more frequently, until finally I was dialing one right after the other, and would hang up the phone more forcefully. When I finally got through the only thing I could think of was finding out who has been on the phone.

3. Waiting for school to get out. Constantly looking at my watch, daydreaming, and could not sit still.

4. Wanting to get home so I could watch a movie on Showtime. Gradually hinting around, kind of pushing my family around telling them they couldn't miss the first of it since it was the best part.

Intervention Proposal: Set of prompts.

1. Every time I find myself starting to get impatient, try to think of alternative things I could do.

Do constructive things
   a. Study, read
   b. Kill time by watching T.V.
   c. Picking up things
2. When people are on time reinforce them.
   Complimenting and thanking
   a. "I'm so glad your here early, now we have time to do (whatever)."
   b. "Thanks for coming on time, now we can get started on this sooner/or get this done faster."

Prompts: Think of things we won't get done unless on schedule. Use prompt ahead of time and immediately reinforce after person is on time.

Treatment: More aware of at what times I would become impatient.

1. Waiting for someone to take my Christmas presents so they could be wrapped. I knew the bus was going to show up in about 5 minutes. I *realized* what I was doing was getting impatient with the older lady who was making out tickets for everyone. Thought to myself that there will be another bus coming in a ½ hour and I still needed to get a few more cards, also that it really wasn't the lady's fault that things were so busy—it's always that way during the holidays. I calmed down and everything was back to the Christmas-spirit again.

2. Waiting for mom to get home from work so we could go shopping, kept looking out the window seeing if I could see her on her way. Noticed I was getting really impatient. Started thinking—"Where is

she—I know she knows I'm waiting for her." Then decided that I really should be finishing up my homework since I had a test coming up in one class and I also had things I needed to complete in my other classes. So I got started on them and before I knew it, mom had showed up and I was one step closer to be caught up on my homework.

Discussion:

I found it really difficult to try to stop being impatient. But the more I am aware of it the easier it is to control by trying to decide on alternative things I could be doing. My project did seem to be a successful one. I'm able to pick up each sign, such as not being able to sit still, starting to get irritable etc., and by thinking of different things I could be doing like finishing my studying, or using prompts to make sure people will try to be on time I can deal with my extreme impatience. I noticed that the time of day is a big factor in this behavior. I'm most impatient towards the end of the day, when I start feeling real run down. Also, I tend to be impatient with one particular person at a given time, therefore, blaming all the lateness on them.

Before I started this project, someone would be late, they'd put me in a bad mood, I'd be mad—nothing would get accomplished and nothing would change. With a behavior such as impatience to work on it really couldn't only be me to cooperate—I had to be sure and prompt others. It was a very hard project because of this reason. I am still a person who gets impatient just like anyone else. The extent has changed in cases like—my phone being busy, waiting for class to get out, and things that it's not possible for me to change. When another person is late when he should be at a particular place I tend to get more impatient—and at these times I am increasingly aware of what is going on and that the best way I should deal with it is through alternatives, reinforcement, and prompts. I am not 100% but now I know what the causes are and interventions that could be used, decreasing the likelihood that I will let myself get as impatient, as I used to be.

UNIT 28

Decreasing Sarcastic Remarks: Report of a Student's Self-Management Project

Project report

A person can modify their actions through a self-management program. If one is not satisfied with their behavior, then that individual needs to take steps toward producing a more desirable behavior. I am not happy with my sarcastic style of speaking. In moderation sarcasm can be humorous, but too much can be boring and self-defeating. A play on another's words can bring yourself desired attention, yet displaying this behavior too often will deter that attention. I would like to decrease my obnoxious terminology. I can gain attention by other means; I can focus my energy into concrete conversations, thus receiving attention from others for my sincerity rather than for the lack thereof. I can attain this goal through the use of a positive reinforcement which is contingent. This process will strengthen my desired behavior, more sincere comments and decrease my undesirable behavior, sarcastic comments.

Method

The subject of this control experiment, obviously, is myself. I am a 16 year old high school senior. I am the youngest of three children and basically, I am a typical "baby" of the family; I have been spoiled, thus I am used to getting my way—any way possible. However, I am aware that certain means of attaining what I want are not always as beneficial to others as they are to myself. Yet I find that I continue on with these behaviors regardless. My main gripe with myself is my sarcasm. I tend to play on others' words and misfortunes to get what I want: attention.

My definition of a sarcastic comment is a twist on another person's comment. This can be done by either reinterpreting what a person says in such a fashion that you create new meaning or creating double connotations. Usually this is done in a blatant manner while people are around to "appreciate" my humor, thus laughing aloud and reinforcing my behavior. Yet at other times the sarcasm is subtle and not everybody catches on, thus making me feel superior. And therefore, I indirectly receive reinforcement by being sly and patting myself on the back. The sarcasm can be sharp and rude, thus insulting the other person. Those around reinforce this behavior by their comments of surprise. At this point, the sarcasm has gone too far—insulting someone to obtain a laugh is not necessary.

To decrease my sarcastic ways, I determined at what points I got out of hand. I carried an index card with me every day for two weeks. I made a note whenever I verbally jabbed someone. I wrote down what I said, to whom, who was around, the time and mood and what was occuring at the onset of the conversation. Through these data I was able to determine when I was most likely to be sarcastic. I became aware of when my sarcasm got to the point of being too much, and I was also shocked to discover just how often I was being sarcastic.

Originally I had planned on using a positive reinforcer to modify my behavior. I still implemented this plan, but I found the reinforcement was not necessary. I experienced what is termed as the intervention effect of the baseline period. Simply counting how often I engaged in my undesirable behavior was enough to decrease it. By observing my own behavior there was a beneficial effect.

During my baseline period it was difficult not to change my behavior. I found that I was most likely to be sarcastic when I felt anger and/or apathy. Most of the time I experience both of these emotions together. If I felt like I just did not care, then my use of "humor" helped to uplift myself. I found that I made jabs at others to boost my own mood. Normally, I was engaged in a "B.S." conversation with my close friends when my sarcasm occurred the most. Usually the comments were directed at my friends. I suppose that I had previously found this type of joking acceptable. When I began to recognize how often it was occurring, I basically became disgusted with myself. I found that I did not need to make rude remarks to my friends to obtain a laugh, nor to gain attention. If I told them that I was not in a good mood, then my friends showed genuine concern: It was them who began joking around to uplift my mood. Not only did I still receive the benefits of humor, but I still was the center of attention. The difference here being that I did not have to act as a jerk to receive this attention.

For the two weeks that I was consciously noting when I had the urge to be sarcastic—I found that as time passed it became much more natural to say something meaningful rather than a sarcastic comment. It was interesting, however, to find that the tendency to say a verbal jab was quite easy. But because I was aware that this was an undesirable behavior I found my reluctance to do such increased immensely. I suppose that through this project I found that being the center of attention is important to me. I'm not sure that I could modify that. However, I did discover that there are more proper means of attaining that attention. There are several forms of humor and being rude to obtain a laugh is not humorous to me anymore.

From a technical standpoint, this project report is only pretty good. It is very sketchy about what the student, Gayle, actually did, and the results are only presented verbally without the actual data. Nonetheless, for Gayle, it was a very important project. At the beginning of the class, she was a very bright but immature and self-centered young woman. Although she continued to be self-centered after completing the project, she had become much more aware of the ways she was acting with her friends and the effects that behavior had on her friends. Both she and her friends felt that she was now much nicer.

This project also clearly demonstrates that a self-management program does not have to be perfect to produce important changes for you. The main point is that when you look at yourself objectively and try to make some changes, good things will usually happen.

UNIT 29

Designing and Conducting a Self-Management Project

It is now time to use the procedures discussed in the analysis of Sarah's program and the students' self-management programs to design your own self-management experiment. In this unit, we go through the steps of designing and conducting a self-management project, using some hypothetical examples. These examples will not necessarily apply to you personally, but basic concepts involved in the examples should be useful for the design of your own project.

Method

Subject

For this project, you will obviously be the subject. You will attempt to analyze and change your own behavior, with the assistance of your instructor, who will act as a consultant. But remember, the project should consist of things that are mainly your *own* ideas.

Target Behavior

The dependent variable for this study will be one of your own responses. Here, you will want to pick out a response that you make that you don't like. That is, it may be a response that gets you in trouble with teachers, parents, or friends (e.g., yelling at your parents); or it could be a response that doesn't get you in trouble but it makes you like yourself less (e.g., overeating or telling small lies). (*At this time, you should pick a behavior that concerns you, but not one that is complex or extremely important. For example, if you find yourself crying a lot when you are alone and don't understand the reason why, you should discuss a problem like that with your parents, school counselor, minister, or some other adult who can help you understand your difficulties.*)

One behavior that frequently causes difficulty for adolescents is speaking without thinking. The exact response involved in such a difficulty can vary tremendously. In defining your target behavior, you will need to specify exactly what you mean by talking without thinking. The behavior you select to work on could be talking back to teachers or parents, making inconsiderate remarks, saying cruel things to friends, and so on; each of these would have different behavioral definitions. Before you can start your self-management project, *you must* have a clear definition of your target behavior that specifies exactly which responses you will count or measure the duration of. After you have selected a target response, write as detailed a behavioral definition as you can, then review it with your instructor.

Recording System

Because you will be collecting data on your own behavior, the process is called "self-recording." *Self-recording* will help you change your behavior in two ways. First of all, it will make you more aware of when you make the response. Often, we don't really realize how many times we make a response during the day. For example, we can make a response such as a cutting remark without being aware of it. We may only vaguely recognize that our friends don't seem to like us as much as they used to. Defining and recording cruel remarks will make a person much more aware of when and how often those responses occur. The person now knows immediately when the response occurs. Because you are trying to change this behavior, the awareness will help you anticipate situations where the behavior might occur so that you can prevent it.

The second major function of *self-recording* is to systematically collect information about the situations in which the behavior occurs, as in the case of the girl who was working on impatience. Another girl, Sharon, was having serious problems with scratching the eczema on her skin until it bled. She was not using her medicine because she did not think that it helped. After collecting a baseline for scratching, Sharon found that she scratched much less on those days she had used the medicine. Her self-management program then involved techniques for increasing the number of times she *appropriately* used her medicine (when using any medicine you should make sure you understand and follow the instructions).

After you have collected a baseline on your target behavior, you need to carefully analyze the records to discover when you made the response and what happened afterward. Then write down some ideas about how to change the behavior. Before starting the self-management procedures, review your ideas with your instructor. Finally, write out the steps of your self-change program. This will help make it very clear what you will be doing to change your behavior.

Sharon solved her scratching problem with the following set of procedures. She was supposed to use the medicine in the morning and in the evening before going to bed. Sharon got two bottles of the lotion; she kept one on her pillow and the second with the towels in the bathroom. At night, when she went to bed, she had to move the medicine to actually get into the bed; this provided a cue to use the medicine. In the morning, while making the bed she simply put the medicine back on the pillow. When she took her shower or washed up in the morning, the second bottle of lotion was with the towels, again providing a cue or prompt to use the lotion. Finally, because the morning was the hardest for her, Sharon taped a reminder and a data sheet to the refrigerator door. In large block letters, it asked, "Did you use your lotion this morning?" The dates were also noted on the data sheet, and Sharon had to check yes or no for that day. Sharon had also discussed the problem with her mother, and her mother had agreed to praise her every morning when she had used the lotion. On her own, Sharon's mother also decided to provide occasional small rewards when Sharon had used the medicine. The project went very well. During the baseline, Sharon had averaged about 10 bad scratching episodes a day. By the end of the self-management project, she was down to 0, and her skin had healed. She continued to use the lotion for another month, then her doctor told her she could stop and the problem did not return. There are a number of points to consider about this project. First, the project procedures were directed at a behavior other than the original target response—that is, using the medicine rather than scratching. The baseline had demonstrated a close relationship between not using the medicine and scratching. As a consequence, it was decided that this was the behavior to change. Second, the main procedures involved using physical cues to increase the number of times Sharon used the medicine. The cues were arranged so that it was very difficult for her to forget her lotion. Finally, her mother was happy to help her and changed from nagging her about scratching (punishment) to praising her for using her medicine (reinforcement).

With this example and the other student reports of self-management projects, you should now have many ideas for ways of changing your own behavior. But remember that all of the concepts and techniques that we have discussed in previous units can be used in a self-management project.

For example, you may wish to negotiate a contract with another person who will help you change a behavior. Sharon could have used a contract with her mother, but the project went smoothly without one. If they had had some difficulty, a contract might have been needed. When you are designing your project, try out many different ideas before selecting the one or two that you will use.

The final point to remember in conducting your self-management project is to be flexible. Carefully monitor the results of your procedures to see if the target behavior is changing. If, after several days or a week, there is no change in your behavior, then you should consider making a change in your procedures. Discuss the progress of your project at least once a week with your instructor.

After you have completed the project, write it up in the same manner as the student reports in Units 25, 26, and 27.

UNIT 30

Smoking as a Self-Management Problem: Psychological Effects and Possible Solutions

Certain behavioral principles govern the responses that occur every day in people's lives. Knowledge of these principles can help people understand why they act the way they do and what they can do to change some of their undesirable behaviors. The following is a discussion of some of the basic principles of behavior and how they might be applied to the problem of smoking.

Smoking is a problem behavior to people who smoke because (1) they often have health problems caused by the smoking, and (2) they almost always find it very difficult to quit smoking. Many nonsmokers also consider smoking a problem because the cigarette smoke of others is offensive to them and is now known to be physically hazardous to them.

When a person studies a behavior, it is necessary to begin by carefully defining that behavior so that there is no confusion about what is meant. Cigarette smoking can be defined as "inhaling cigarette smoke." But what about people who sit near a smoker and breathe the smoke—are they smoking? Of course not. But you can see that it is necessary to define the behavior precisely. Perhaps the definition should include putting the cigarette to the lips, drawing smoke into the mouth, and exhaling.

It is also useful to measure how much or how often the behavior occurs. The measure of smoking behavior could be the number of cigarettes smoked, the amount of time spent smoking or the total number of puffs taken on all cigarettes smoked. Before beginning a program to change a behavior, one should keep a record of this measure for a period of time. This information is the baseline, and it is useful in planning a program for behavior change as well as in determining whether or not any change has occurred.

In developing a program for changing a behavior or for preventing it from occurring, it is helpful to know what kinds of things or events may be responsible for that behavior occurring in the first place. Some psychologists believe that the frequency with which a behavior occurs depends on what happens immediately after it (the subsequent stimulus). If a behavior occurs more frequently than it had before the introduction of the subsequent stimulus, then the behavior is said to have been *reinforced*. A reinforcer (1) happens immediately after a response (behavior), (2) increases the likelihood that the behavior will occur again, and (3) is something the person seeks and cannot get easily elsewhere.

Positive reinforcement is something pleasant that occurs after a behavior and increases the probability that it will occur again. What might be some of the positive reinforcers that are responsible for smoking behavior? Some people feel more relaxed after smoking a cigarette. If relaxation follows immediately after smoking behavior occurs, and it increases the frequency of smoking, then it is a reinforcer. Also, nicotine is a drug that goes into circulation in the body very quickly while a person is smoking. It appears to have some physiological effects that people report as rewarding and pleasurable.

For many people, however, smoking is not followed by greater relaxation. Other events must be responsible for the behavior. Many people, especially young people, get attention from their peers for smoking. They may have been relatively deprived of attention before they tried smoking; when smoking, they may have found that some of their classmates talked to them and interacted with them more often.

Some young people may start smoking for slightly different reasons. Suppose that their peers tease and embarrass them because they are not "grown up" enough or "man" (woman) enough to smoke. They may decide to start smoking just to prove themselves to these peers. If they start smoking and the peers stop their harassment, then chances are they will continue to smoke. This is an example of negative reinforcement. Negative reinforcement always involves removal of an aversive or unpleasant event, resulting in an increased probability that the behavior preceding such removal will occur. In addition, the peer group may now become more positive to the person because the person is smoking. So there would be positive peer reinforcement for the behavior.

A number of other types of events can influence behavior. Punishment and extinction are two that decrease the probability that a behavior will occur. Suppose that Jenny is part of a group of students who smoke.

The group reinforces smoking behavior with social interaction. But now Jenny decides that she would like to be friends with Joe, too. Joe is a nonsmoker, and he dislikes smoking by others. Joe refuses to talk to Jenny whenever he sees her with a cigarette, so Jenny gradually quits smoking when she's around Joe. Joe's behavior of ignoring Jenny for smoking is an example of extinction. *Extinction* means the withholding of reinforcement, and it usually results in decreased rate of that response. It is often a successful way to get rid of problem behaviors.

Punishment refers to the presentation of an aversive event or the removal of a pleasant one. Punishment decreases the probability that a behavior will occur, but it may also lead to a general disruption of behavior, and it thus should not be used when another procedure (e.g., extinction) could be used for the same problem. Jenny's parents might punish her if she were to smoke at home. They could take away some privileges, such as staying out late on weekends; they could "ground" her for a week or take away her allowance for a while. Or they might even physically slap her. Jenny probably would not smoke at home again, but she might also become very angry, yell at her family and other people as well, or go to her room and sulk. These are examples of some kinds of negative behavior that can result from punishment.

It seems as if certain situations are associated with reinforcement of a behavior, while others signal punishment or extinction. The peer group that reinforces smoking (positively) is called a *discriminative stimulus* (S^D) for smoking behavior. On the other hand, parents, teachers, and nonsmoking classmates do not reinforce smoking. They are called S-deltas (S^Δ's). Events that are associated with reinforcement are S^D's. Those that are associated with *no* reinforcement are S^Δ's.

Changing smoking (or any other) behavior could be accomplished by arranging one's environment so that those events or people that usually serve as signals for that behavior to occur are not present. Similarly, one could arrange to be in situations that are associated with a lack of reinforcement for the behavior.

Changing a behavior can also be accomplished by arranging the consequences so that reinforcement does not occur for that behavior. This procedure can be made even more effective by arranging for other behaviors to occur that can provide similar reinforcers. Attention and peer interaction, as well as a number of other reinforcers that people receive for smoking, can also be received for participation in such other activities as sports, music, and hobbies. But many young people feel that they are not qualified or talented enough to engage in these activities. However, the skills or abilities necessary can be developed. A process called *shaping* involves reinforcement of closer and closer approximations to a "target" behavior or goal. Playing a piece of music on the piano is an example of a behavior that is shaped. At first, the notes are played very slowly and many mistakes are made. But improvement in playing is reinforced by the sound of the music produced. With practice, anyone can learn and can enjoy making music.

The same process occurs in learning to serve a tennis ball. When a player makes the right moves, he/she is reinforced with a good serve. Soon, the person learns which moves are responsible for good serves. It is important to remember that no one knows how to do such activities who hasn't learned them in just this way. Shaping can also be used in developing skills that could help an individual to get an interesting (and profitable) job.

People who find that they have undesirable behaviors that they would like to change can do so by using the aforementioned principles of behavior. They can avoid situations that promote (reinforce) the behaviors, arrange negative consequences such as extinction or punishment, or develop skills to substitute for the unwanted behavior. Often they find that they can receive even more desirable consequences for the newly developed skills.

One way to employ the principles in a program for behavior change is to develop a *behavioral contract*. The contract is a written agreement between the person who desires to change his/her behavior and another person or group of persons. It should include a clear statement of the goal of the program, the specific behavior to be changed, and the consequences for complying and for not complying with the program. A person who desires to stop smoking could develop a contract with a group of nonsmoking friends. The goal would be smoking no cigarettes at all. A definition of the behavior of smoking should be made. The ultimate goal could be divided into several steps, such as reduction of the number smoked per day by 2, then by 4, and so on. The consequences could be anything from ignoring the person when smoking occurs, and providing attention at all other times, to fining the person $.50 for each cigarette smoked above the limit for the day. A large reward could be specified for when the ultimate goal is reached (perhaps a trip to a movie or dinner at a special restaurant, paid for by the others with the fines collected).

Every contract, of course, will have to be developed by those involved, using consequences that will be effective for the participants. It should be modified if it does not seem to be producing changes in the desired direction. When these conditions are met, contracting can be a simple and direct method of employing behavioral principles for successful behavior change.

Study Guide

1. Smoking is a problem behavior because:

   a. _____

   b. _____

2. List three possible positive reinforcers for smoking.

   a. _____

   b. _____

   c. _____

3. Escape from peer teasing about not smoking could be a

   _____ reinforcer for smoking.

4. Situations or groups of people that have been associated with smoking in the past are _____ stimuli for smoking.

5. One method of decreasing smoking is to avoid

   _____ stimuli for smoking.

6. A person who wants to stop smoking can develop a behavioral

   _____ with nonsmoking friends.

UNIT 31

Stopping Smoking: Report of a Student's Self-Management Project

The following report describes how a young man who was a student in one of the classes used these procedures to eliminate his smoking behavior. As you read the report, make an outline of the procedures he used.

Subject: Rob
Program: Termination of smoking behavior

Through this designed self-control project, I hope to establish a zero frequency smoking behavior under all antecedent conditions. The antecedents to my smoking behavior encompass every situation except sleeping. I wish to terminate my smoking behavior for I have noticed my physical deterioration. I wheeze, gurgle, cough and grow winded easily. Another dominant factor is the cost involved in supporting my smoking behavior. My finances are dwindling and I'm finding it increasingly difficult to obtain the needed dollar for a pack of cigarettes.

Baseline. To establish my average daily number of cigarettes smoked, I collected a baseline on the target behavior for two weeks. I recorded each cigarette smoked on a daily note card prior to my lighting the cigarette. Gathering the baseline had a temporary intervention effect but in a matter of four days those effects had stabilized to a regular level. Data was collected and an average established. The target behavior averaged at twenty cigarettes a day, slightly more on the weekends and slightly less during the week.

Intervention. I chose to use shaping as the base for my intervention plan. I would immediately drop my average from twenty cigarettes a day to ten a day. This was my point of departure. I would smoke one less cigarette each consecutive day until after ten days I would acquire my zero frequency smoking behavior. In my case, a monetary reinforcement schedule would supply the most potent reinforcer. Terry, my brother, whom I see every morning, evening, and a few scattered classes throughout the day, was the obvious choice to uphold this portion of the contract. I gave him twelve dollars to dole out to me fifty cents each morning if I had smoked that day's allotted number of cigarettes. If I had not met the days criterion, Terry would pocket the fifty cents. To counteract temptation, each morning Terry also gave me that days allotted number of cigarettes so I wouldn't be carrying around a full pack. The intervention plan was designed to continue reinforcement for 2 weeks after I had attained a zero frequency smoking behavior. As I informed friends of my plans to quit smoking, social reinforcement was spontaneously added to the intervention plan. Friends refrained from smoking in my presence, some tried themselves to quit and all applauded my progress.

Self-Contract

Other: October 22   Self: Rob
                                                               Other: Terry
  Goal: To attain a zero frequency smoking behavior

Agreement
  Self: I agree to smoke only ten cigarettes this day, nine cigarettes tomorrow, eight the next day, etc., until I reach a frequency of zero cigarettes a day.

Consequences
  Self: If contract is kept I will acquire fifty cents each morning. If contract is broken I will forfeit fifty cents each morning to Terry.
  Other: If contract is kept Terry will award me with fifty cents and praise my progress. If contract is broken Terry will pocket the fifty cents for himself.

Exceptions
  Only exception will be if program is revised and contract revision necessary.
Review Date: November 14

Results
  My intervention plan went quite well for the first six days. Immediately dropping to ten cigarettes on the first day posed no problem. On

the seventh day of intervention, however, I found myself at a plateau. I smoked five cigarettes when the days allotment was only four so Terry gained fifty cents. The eighth day, again attempting to smoke only four cigarettes, I could not gain control over my behavior so I was out another fifty cents. The ninth day went the same and I found it necessary to revise my intervention plan.

Revision

I found the shaping schedule to be too directed. I reasoned that if I could smoke only four cigarettes and maintain that level for five days I would then have attained enough control over my behavior to drop to a zero frequency level. Reinforcement was to continue in the same manner under the new schedule so a contract revision was unnecessary.

Results

The revised intervention plan was a success. Once the first day of the revision was successfully completed, the following four days went smoothly. I then directly dropped to the zero frequency target behavior and had no problem maintaining that level. The reinforcement continued for ten days sustaining my new non-smoking behavior.

Evaluation

The designed self-control project was highly successful as illustrated by my new zero frequency smoking behavior. The choice of reinforcement was a primary factor in this success. I've been miserly since I can remember. Losing fifty cents a day for performing an undesirable act (smoking), is as foolish as flushing the money down the toilet. I have also come to believe that the social reinforcement gained from my peers had a great effect on my behavior. Friends constantly asked how I was doing on my project and rather than lie, I found the only alternative to be to continue on the program. The procedures I followed probably wouldn't work for every person, but for me the method brought success.

Maintenance

Once a zero frequency smoking behavior has been reached it is necessary to continue the monetary reinforcement until control over the behavior has been established. It's preposterous to conceive of indefinite monetary reinforcement schedule so another means of maintenance is required. Social reinforcement is the answer. Keeping friends informed of your accomplishment brings the praise needed for future maintenance. *You can truly be proud of yourself for quitting the cigarette habit and this pride ultimately aids in maintaining your new behavior in the future.*

You have been taught a number of ways to change your behavior and the behavior of other people. Now imagine that you have a problem with smoking, you smoke, and you would like to stop. Further suppose that some of your friends smoke but do not want to stop. Finally, your parents know you smoke and would like you to stop, but you and your parents are not getting along very well. Now design a program to change your behavior and solve the problems. Be sure to analyze the variables that might be influencing your smoking behaviors and how they might be changed to help you stop smoking.

When you have finished your analyses of the first problem, work on the following situation. You do not smoke but some of your friends do. Your friends often offer you cigarettes, but you really don't want to smoke. Suggest ways that you could refuse to smoke while still keeping your friends.

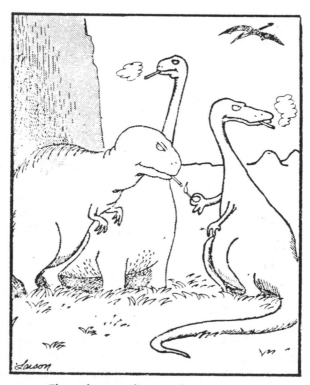

The real reason dinosaurs became extinct.
The Far Side cartoon reprinted by permission of Chronicle Features, San Francisco.

UNIT 32

Alcohol and Self-Management: Some Information about Alcohol

There is probably no other issue that causes more problems between youths and adults (especially adolescents and their parents) than the question of drinking alcoholic beverages. Usually, the conflict can be clearly, if somewhat crudely, summarized by the following accusative question: You drink—why can't I? Equally often, the adult does not have a good answer and resorts to threats of dire consequences and punishments if the youth does drink. Frequently, such an exchange results in an angry argument between the youth and his/her parents. The final result often is that the youth concludes that the adult is a hypocrite and that the reasons for not drinking are not worth considering. Such an outcome is unfortunate because it is likely to lead to more conflict and potentially damaging drinking patterns.

Is there a good answer to the question, "If you drink, why can't I?" One might point out that not all behaviors modelled by adults are good things to do; that, however, is probably a cop-out. The best answer is a straightforward but complex one. Alcohol is a pleasurable but potentially dangerous drug. It influences how you behave and can lead individuals to act in ways that they might not ordinarily wish to. It requires both physiological and psychological maturity to drink pleasurably, safely, and responsibly. Of course, such maturity does not magically occur with reaching the legal drinking age. It comes rather from developing the self-control skills we have discussed and practiced throughout this manual. It comes with the recognition that drinking to get drunk never has been and never will be cool. It comes with the recognition that escaping problems with an alcohol-induced euphoria does not solve those problems. In short, many adults, as well as youths, should not drink. The objective of this section of the workbook is not to teach you that alcohol is bad and that you should never drink (you may reach those conclusions on your own, but that is not our purpose in writing this section). Rather, our concern is to provide you with the facts about drinking so that when you are older, you may make a reasoned judgment about whether you wish to drink, how much to drink, and under what circumstances to drink. *We strongly recommend that individuals below the legal drinking age should not consume alcoholic beverages.* If, however, you do drink either occasionally or frequently, there are a number of things you should know about the effects of alcohol and how to control your drinking rate.

Let us begin the discussion of drinking by examining the effects of alcohol on the central nervous system. When we speak of the central nervous system we are mainly concerned with the brain. Neurophysiologists, neuroanatomists, biochemists, psychologists, and others have studied the parts and functions of the brain for many years, and while there is much that is not understood, some useful distinctions can be made. First, the most recently developed part of the brain is called the neocortex, or the cerebral cortex (not all animals' brains have a neocortex), and it seems to be involved in what is loosely labeled "higher intellectual functioning." Such activities as talking, thinking, remembering, and the like seem to be a function of the cerebral cortex. Another important section of the brain is the midbrain and hypothalamus. These areas are related mostly to the regulation of consummatory behavior (eating and drinking) and most emotional behavior. Finally, there is the cerebellum, which mostly controls balance and coordination. There are many other important areas and functions of the brain, but alcohol affects these areas primarily.

The brain operates largely as a function of many small biochemical reactions. Alcohol is an organic chemical compound that interferes with the biochemical functioning of the brain. Alcohol is called a *depressant* drug because it depresses, or slows, the body's functioning. As a consequence, when there are light to moderate amounts of alcohol in the blood, many people report that alcoholic beverages are relaxing. The alcohol slows the biochemical functioning of the brain and reduces muscle tension. If that were the extent of alcohol's effect on the body, then there would be less to worry about. Unfortunately, as alcohol accumulates in the bloodstream, it increasingly interferes with the body's functioning; eventually, death can occur at high enough blood alcohol concentrations. Even at lower blood alcohol concentrations, the alcohol can severely interfere with the brain's operation: loss of balance, slurring speech, and impairment of the ability to reason. For those reasons, it is extremely important for anyone who drinks to be aware of the progressive effects of alcohol. The term "blood alcohol concentration" (BAC) refers to the amount of alcohol concentration in circulation in the bloodstream.

In the following discussion, BAC is recorded in terms of milligrams of alcohol per 100 milliliters of blood, which is translated into milligrams percent (mg%). Sometimes, BAC is reported as a decimal percentage such as .10%. This figure is equivalent to 100 mg%. As indicated earlier, the effects of alcohol on the drinker are determined by the amount of alcohol in the bloodstream.

- At 20 mg% light and moderate drinkers begin to feel some effects. This is the approximate BAC after one drink.
- At 40 mg%, most people begin to feel relaxed.
- At 60 mg%, judgment is somewhat impaired; people are less able to make rational decisions about their capabilities (e.g., to drive).
- At 80 mg%, there is definite impairment of muscle coordination and driving skills—legally drunk in some states.
- At 100 mg%, there is clear deterioration of reaction time and control—legally drunk in most states.
- At 120 mg%, vomiting occurs unless this level is reached slowly.
- At 150 mg%, balance and movement are impaired. This BAC level means that the equivalent of 1 half-pint of whiskey is circulating in the bloodstream.
- At 300 mg%, many people lose consciousness.
- At 400 mg%, most people lose consciousness; some die.
- At 450 mg%, breathing stops; death results.

How alcohol affects a person and the rate that alcohol accumulates in the bloodstream are determined by three factors: how much the person weighs, how fast the person drinks, and (obviously) how much he/she drinks. The next set of tables indicate the BAC accumulated as a function of the number of drinks, body weight, and time. In these tables, one drink stands for the amount of alcohol in one 12-ounce bottle of beer, one 4-ounce glass of table wine, or one 1-ounce drink of distilled spirits (hard liquor such as gin, vodka, or scotch). As different as these drinks may seem, they all contain the same amount of alcohol. The table presented below is called a "blood alcohol concentration guide."

Blood Alcohol Concentration: A Guide

Body Weight	Number of drinks									
	1	2	3	4	5	6	7	8	9	10
100	.029	.058	.088	.117	.146	.175	.204	.233	.262	.290
120	.024	.048	.073	.097	.121	.145	.170	.194	.219	.243
140	.021	.042	.063	.083	.104	.125	.146	.166	.187	.208
160	.019	.037	.055	.073	.091	.109	.128	.146	.164	.182
180	.017	.033	.049	.065	.081	.097	.113	.130	.146	.162
200	.015	.029	.044	.058	.073	.087	.102	.117	.131	.146
220	.014	.027	.040	.053	.067	.080	.093	.106	.119	.133
240	.012	.024	.037	.048	.061	.073	.085	.097	.109	.122

Alcohol is burned up by your body at .015% per hour, as follows:

Number of hours since starting first drink	1	2	3	4	5	6
Percent alcohol burned up	.015	.030	.045	.060	.075	.090

Example: 180-pound man—8 drinks in 4 hours is .130% on the chart. Subtract .060% burned up in 4 hours. BAC equals .070%—*judgment impaired*.

Using this table, it is possible to calculate the BAC from consuming a particular number of drinks over a given period of time. Once the BAC has been estimated, it is possible to predict how the alcohol will affect behavior. Try to estimate the BAC and how a person would be affected in the following situations. For the exercise, use your own weight in figuring the BAC. Because the table is in 20-pound intervals, you should round off to the nearest weight in the table.

1. The individual has had three beers in 45 minutes. What is the BAC, and is it safe for this person to drive a car?

2. Two friends have been drinking steadily for the last 3 hours and have finished a pint of vodka (16 ounces). What are their BACs (assume that each person drinks 8 ounces), and can they trust their own judgment?

3. A person had two glasses of wine an hour ago. What is his/her BAC now?

4. A female acquaintance (assume she weighs 120) has had four glasses of wine in the past 2 hours. Now she wants to drive home. What is her BAC, and is it safe for her to drive her car?

5. A male (weight 160) has just finished a six-pack in the last 2 hours and wants to go water-skiing. What is his BAC, and is it safe for him to water-ski?

6. If a person wished to keep BAC at or below 60 mg%, how many drinks can he/she have in an hour? in 3 hours?

Without sounding moralistic, after carefully reviewing the literature on adolescent drinking, we can honestly make only one recommendation to you concerning drinking alcoholic beverages—*don't*! If we had found evidence that consumption of alcohol can be of long-term benefit to the adolescent, we would not make such a strong statement, but there is none. Regular consumption of more than very small amounts of alcohol is a clear example of a self-control problem. The immediate consequences of drinking may be somewhat pleasurable but the long-term consequences of adolescent drinking are extremely negative.

Study Guide

1. A frequent topic of arguments between parents and adolescents is

_____ alcoholic beverages.

2. Alcohol is a potentially _____
drug.

3. Escaping a problem in an alcohol-induced euphoria does not

_____ that problem.

4. The brain functions through many small

_____ reactions.

5. Alcohol is an organic chemical compound that

_____ with the biochemical

_____ of the brain.

6. Alcohol can have _____ effects
on behavior.

7. In the presence of alcohol, balance is

_____, speech is

_____, and the ability to reason

is _____.

8. The research on drinking clearly indicates that adolescents should

    _____ drink alcoholic beverages.

UNIT 33

Alcohol and Self-Management: Some Techniques for Changing Drinking Habits

This unit is designed to provide you with some information about how drinking habits can be changed. We do not recommend that adolescents try to change their own drinking habits without assistance. The first step for anyone who recognizes that he/she has a problem with alcohol is to seek assistance. Teenage alcoholism is a steadily growing problem. Often, the adolescent who is drinking too much feels that adults will only punish or condemn such behavior and not provide assistance in solving the problems. This is not true! Many adults are truly interested in helping adolescents with drinking problems. Friends of individuals having drinking problems need to encourage and help that person find people who can provide the needed assistance. (One organization that can help the person directly or can help the person find help is Alcoholics Anonymous. Further, most communities will have an agency designed to assist people with alcohol problems.)

Drinking beverages is a widely practiced social activity by youths. Some adolescents don't drink at all, while others may drink frequently, and/or drink large amounts at one time. Drinking alcohol can be a behavior problem because (1) it can be dangerous to health, (2) it may cause problems in social and family life, and/or (3) it may create problems at work or at school. Assuming that a person is having difficulty with alcohol, what can that individual do about those problems?

Although problems with alcohol may be more difficult to solve than some of the self-management problems discussed earlier, the same basic approach can be pursued with great success. To review, the essential steps in self-management are (1) define the target behavior; (2) record a baseline of the target behavior; (3) analyze the situations in which the target behavior occurs; (4) determine the consequences of the behavior that may be reinforcing it; (5) design a set of self-management procedures to change the behavior; finally, (6) continually evaluate how well the procedures are working, and change them if necessary. In this section, we illustrate how self-management techniques can be used to change a person's drinking habits.

The problem behavior must first be defined in order to study and change it. The definition in this case might be drinking any type of alcoholic beverage. But suppose someone put alcohol in punch at a party without anyone knowing it. Should drinking the punch be considered a problem behavior that needs to be changed? Perhaps the definition should include something about the person being aware that he/she is drinking alcohol. Because the tables used for calculating BAC define one drink as a bottle of beer, 4 ounces of wine, or 1 ounce of hard liquor, those measures should be used in the definition of drinking behavior. For instance, if someone is given a tomato juice drink known to have 2 ounces of vodka in it (commonly called a Bloody Mary), such a beverage would not only be classified as an example of the target behavior, but it would also count as two drinks.

Some drinking may be considered problem drinking, while other drinking may not. A person who only drinks one beer every Friday night probably would not consider drinking a problem. However, a person who drinks enough beer on a Friday night to black out, wake up Saturday morning with a hangover, and argue with his/her parents about drinking may or may not define drinking as a problem, but clearly it is.

The first step in changing a problem behavior is to collect a baseline to find out how much it occurs, with whom, where, and when. This can be done by keeping a record of every alcoholic drink that is consumed. How much alcohol is in the drink, what time and day it is, where the drinker is, and who else is there should be written down before taking a drink. This procedure is called self-monitoring. The record should be kept for a week or 2 before the person tries to change the behavior. The information collected is used as a starting point (baseline) from which to improve.

It is important to look at what happens immediately *after* the behavior because this influences the initial behavior. It is thus necessary to examine what occurs after a drink is taken. There may be some positive things, such as becoming more relaxed, feeling more accepted by peers, or losing some shyness. All of these are positive consequences and may increase the number of times the drinking occurs. If the consequences increase the frequency of the original behavior, they are called reinforcers. Some negative things may also be experienced as the result of drinking. Examples are hangovers, long-term health problems, and family problems. Because these also occur after the behavior, they may influence drinking. You might think they would decrease the frequency of the original behavior (by punishing it). However, as we learned in the section on self-management, immediate consequences are often more powerful than delayed ones. Again, in the case of drinking, the reason the negative consequences of drinking do not usually influence drinking behavior as much as the positive consequences is that the positive consequences are more immediate. Relaxation, praise given from friends, euphoria, and so on, are all felt before a hangover and long before health problems.

It is also important to look at things that occur *before* the problem behavior. It may be that the problem behavior occurs in certain situations only. Once these situations are identified, ways can be found to deal with them. The specific situation that is present before the behavior is called the discriminative stimulus (S^D). Examples would be other people the individual is drinking with, the place, or the specific time of the day or week. For example, a person may discover that he/she only overdrinks when in the company of one particular individual. Then the program for changing problem drinking would concentrate on modifying the interactions with that individual.

There are many other things that can be done systematically to change problem drinking behavior. An important factor is the speed of drinking—how fast a person drinks. As the table in Unit 32 demonstrates, how quickly drinks are consumed influences the amount of alcohol that is in the bloodstream. The amount of alcohol in the bloodstream determines how the person will act or how drunk the person is. If six beers are consumed in 1 hour, the person will be more intoxicated than if the drinking was spread over 3 hours. An examination of the baseline record may show that a person does not drink very often, but when he/she does it results in intoxication. It may be further determined that the person overdrinks because he/she drinks too fast. If so, the self-management program should be designed to slow down the drinking rate. One way to slow down drinking is to take smaller sips. If a beer is usually finished in six gulps, making the sips half as large (twelve gulps per beer), while keeping the time between sips the same results in slower drinking. Another method is alternating alcoholic drinks and soft drinks without alcohol. This technique gives the individual something in the hand, but it cuts down on the amount of alcohol consumed. Such alternation is useful when a person attends a party at which the drinking will continue for a long time. Other ways to slow down drinking include drinking mixed drinks instead of straight shots and drinking drinks that the person dislikes rather than drinking drinks the person favors.

Because the events that occur immediately after the behavior affect the future frequency of those behaviors, it is important to look at what happens during and after drinking. For example, if Bob's friends only accept him if he drinks a lot, he might want to find friends that will accept him without drinking. If he spends time with people who encourage him not to drink, he will probably drink less. If Sue drinks because it relaxes her, she can try to find other ways to relax. Some of the various ways people have found to relax are yoga, meditation, or simply lying down and shutting their eyes for 15 minutes. Any *desirable effect* that people get by drinking alcohol *can* be obtained by another *less dangerous and more enjoyable method.*

Events occurring before a behavior is performed are also important in a behavior change program. Changing the discriminative stimuli may make behavior change easier. For example, if Janet finds she always gets drunk with Steve, Mary, and Joe on Friday nights riding around in her car, changing any of these may lead to less drinking. If she goes out with different people or does something besides driving around in the car, the drinking pattern might change. She could also choose to do something on Friday night that is incompatible with drinking—that is, an activity that is difficult to do while you drink. Avoiding situations where overdrinking is encouraged (such as "chugging" contests) is also important.

The ideas concerning changing drinking behavior have been presented to illustrate the factors that influence drinking by young people. It is important to reiterate that we cannot recommend the use of alcoholic beverages by adolescents. Further, a person who discovers that he/she has difficulties with drinking should not try to solve these difficulties by him/herself. The abuse of alcohol is a complex psychological problem, so the person should certainly seek help.

Study Guide

Rather than providing a regular study guide for this unit, we want you to prepare for the class discussion by trying to answer the following broad questions.

1. Why do some adolescents drink?

2. Why, of those who drink, do some have very serious problems with alcohol?

3. Can you express your ideas about the difficulties with alcohol in terms of stimulus control factors and positive and negative reinforcers for drinking?

4. How could you help someone who has a drinking problem?

Epilogue

In the last few units, we have discussed two major self-control problems: drinking alcoholic beverages and smoking. While these are important problems, we wish to emphasize that the techniques of applied psychology and self-management presented in the book can best be used to deal with the small everyday problems. If you understand these concepts and procedures, they can be then used to make your interactions with friends, family, and significant others much more positive. We hope that the manual has helped you understand and change your behavior in even some smaller ways. Finally, it should be clear that science relates to the conduct of our daily lives, and we hope that some of you will decide to pursue a career in science.